Designing and analysing questionnaires and surveys: a manual for health professionals and administrators

Designing and analysing questionnaires and surveys

A manual for health professionals and administrators

CHRIS J. JACKSON
University of Surrey

AND

ADRIAN FURNHAM
University College London

W
WHURR PUBLISHERS LTD
LONDON AND PHILADELPHIA

© 2000 Whurr Publishers
First published 2000 by
Whurr Publishers Ltd
19b Compton Terrace, London N1 2UN, England and
325 Chestnut Street, Philadelphia PA 19106, USA

Reprinted 2001

All rights reserved. No part of this publication may be reproduced, stored in a retrieval system, or transmitted in any form or by any means, electronic, mechanical, photocopying, recording or otherwise without the prior permission of Whurr Publishers Limited.

This publication is sold subject to the conditions that it shall not, by way of trade or otherwise, be lent, resold, hired out, or otherwise circulated without the publisher's prior consent in any form of binding or cover other than that in which it is published and without a similar condition including this condition being imposed upon any subsequent purchaser.

British Library Cataloguing in Publication Data
A catalogue record for this book is available from the British Library.

ISBN 1 86156 072 9

Printed and bound in the UK by Athenaeum Press Ltd, Gateshead, Tyne & Wear

Contents

Introduction	vii

Part 1 Background principles — 1

1	The basic rationale	3
2	Determining objectives and hypotheses	18
3	Under what circumstances should the survey be undertaken?	27
4	Researching the problem	52

Part 2 The general survey design — 63

5	An overview of the design	65
6	Choosing between postal and interview surveys	73
7	Obtaining the right size and type of sample	92

Part 3 Survey and questionnaire formats — 97

8	Generating the items	99
9	Writing the survey	111

Part 4 Evaluating the items — 135

10	The pilot study	137

Part 5 Analysing the results — 151

11	Analysing data from surveys	153

Part 6 The report — 183

12	Presenting the survey results	185
13	Evaluating reports	191
14	Example reports together with introductory critiques	198

References	277

Introduction

Some professions are well known for their investment in survey research. For example, in advertising and politics there is a clear need to know what people are thinking: why people buy certain products rather than others; how people intend to vote; how much they trust certain politicians; and how much certain policies are liked. Hotels and airlines, indeed nearly all service industries, attempt to 'poll' their customers to find out their sources of satisfaction and dissatisfaction. They know that they have to be, as well as have to be seen to be, responsive to the needs of their clients. Chances are that virtually all the readers of this book have been asked to take part in a survey at some point in their lives. How comfortable was the airline? What is your opinion of this fizzy drink compared to that one? Who would you vote for if there was a general election next week? Open a newspaper and you will be able to read endless articles providing you with questionnaire and survey results: 'survey shows pay has risen by less than the cost of inflation'; '45% of undergraduate women claim to have been harassed on campus'; and '11% of primary school children admit to being offered drugs'. The media tends to sensationalize the results of surveys and can therefore undermine the serious intent of some of the Researchers. Going behind the headlines will generally show you that serious Researchers have conducted a survey or questionnaire to obtain accurate information in terms of attitudes, beliefs, values, motives and/or facts. Organizations know that the investment in information collection pays dividends because it results in better quality decision making. Unfortunately, this may not always be true within the health professions. In fact, there can often be resistance towards research, although of course there are also many examples of excellence.

The most significant reasons why survey research is *not* conducted and *not* put into practice within the health professions include:

(a) Lack of knowledge, skills and technical training: many people working as health professionals simply have not heard about relevant research, find access to libraries difficult and do not have the expertise to evaluate and apply findings.
(b) Lack of belief in the research: many health professionals are not convinced by the quality of the research they see. They may pour scorn on the idea through mistaken beliefs about the extent to which people lie. Also they may not understand sampling theory, believing that one has to survey all users to gain an accurate picture.
(c) Lack of permission: many are not allowed to implement new ideas by introducing changes that appear to be useful in the light of research evidence. For example, the idea of sampling patients' satisfaction with treatment and/or service can provide valuable feedback to those organizations that are responsive to patients' needs. On the other hand, it may be hard for senior management to rise to the challenge, since there may be criticisms of the way things are done at present.
(d) Lack of commitment: many health professionals have little incentive or reward to introduce changes. Many find that they are not encouraged and there are few role models from whom inspiration can be drawn.
(e) Lack of resources to plan, execute and analyse the study. The amount of money needed to conduct a survey is often not that large, but money is nonetheless necessary. Without adequate resourcing, the research cannot be done.

The fundamental aim of this book is to provide accessible, detailed good practice guidelines that also address the political and ethical problems of conducting surveys within the health professions. We intend to demystify, educate and provide the kind of practical tips that will make the process as straightforward as possible. To achieve these ends, we believe that we have gone beyond many of the standard texts on the subject by introducing informed opinion, useful examples, sections on how things should be done in practice as opposed to in theory, and hopefully the occasional more light-hearted section to add some humour to the book. In short, we have set out to produce a fresh and original book that does not draw heavily on established texts.

Introduction

We also try to address, albeit indirectly, the lack of incentive that is all too often found in collecting quality data that can bring about useful change. By carrying out high-quality work, those involved in a survey project, including the readers of the final report, are likely to be excited and interested in implementing the valid and useful conclusions that are drawn from the data. Following high-quality methods will provide the kind of unarguable evidence that will impress even the most negative decision maker. All our examples are drawn from the health sector to illustrate the points we make.

Two types of survey are commonly commissioned within the health professions. First, surveys are conducted on patients and patients' health and, second, surveys on staff are used to collect accurate information about actual work practice and attitudes towards work practice. Such surveys are often carried out by health professionals and health administrators. However, it is fair to say that many health professionals have developing administrative interests, and many health administrators have medical responsibilities. As a result, this book draws no distinction between these two roles and therefore provides a unique perspective on survey design methods within the health sector. The following examples are typical of the ways in which surveys and questionnaires are used within the health professions:

- Clinical psychologists are interested in assessing patients' mood after a certain type of operation or specialized treatment (chemotherapy, homeopathy, etc.).
- Doctors send out a questionnaire to patients to collect information about side-effects from a certain type of drug.
- Medical staff need to design a checklist of comatose patients' symptoms that can be completed by a nurse.
- Psychiatrists wish to design a questionnaire to measure a psychiatric condition that can be used by non-specialists.
- Hospital management are interested in determining demographic details of patients in the locality (e.g. sex, age, education, self-reported health, etc.).
- Local health managers are interested in determining the major reasons why out-patients do not turn up for appointments.
- Health employers may wish to monitor the sex and race of staff to determine if they meet equal opportunities legislation.
- Hospital management may commission a survey to determine what patients think of current work practices.

- A health union is interested in determining levels of stress experienced by staff.
- The head of nursing may wish to determine what is the greatest source of dissatisfaction to nurses within a particular hospital.
- A catering manager may wish to determine what customers think about the food served in the canteen.

These are just a few examples of the ways in which surveys and questionnaires are used to provide key information to decision makers within the health professions. Well designed, administered and analysed, they can show who believes what, why people behave in a particular way, and what their hopes and expectations are.

This book will, we hope, appeal to three types of person whether they are wearing their health professional or administrator 'hats'. First, the 'keen amateurs' within the health professions who would like to conduct a survey but do not know where to begin. These best practice guidelines will, we hope, be of great benefit to these people. Second, the book is aimed at those non-experts within the health profession who *commission* a survey. Such people will find the book useful in helping them choose between tendered offers and to review the quality of the survey information that has been gathered. We hope that this book will help these people become educated consumers. They can thus determine if a project proposal covers the relevant ground and, later on, make an informed opinion about whether or not the conclusions that others have drawn have been soundly made. Third, the book is aimed at providing an easy practitioner's perspective of survey design to introduce *students* to this subject area. Students tend to have one of two reactions to learning about surveys: they are either bored or fearful. The practical and tailored advice within this book addresses both of these issues and provides a firm foundation for the student to move on to more advanced texts.

The book is designed to be either read in its entirety or dipped into. Although it is often a good idea to read all of a book so that a complete perspective is achieved, it is recognized that many readers simply do not have the time for such luxuries. For readers who wish to read certain sections only, the fast entry diagrams at the end of this section are a good place to start.

Introduction

Having stated the aim of the book, it is probably fair to say what the book does not aim to do. We do not seek to provide the unqualified with instant competence. Such people must understand that survey design can be difficult and without foresight is rarely straightforward. To those who wish to conduct a survey with no past experience and who believe they already have the skills, there is just one simple message: *read this book thoroughly*. Otherwise the survey will be flawed and the results poorly received when the work is reviewed by experts.

Here are just a few of the typical mistakes made by inexperienced survey designers:

- Unethical studies that result in the Researcher being disciplined, struck off or imprisoned (e.g. for asking inappropriate questions, breaching anonymity, selling confidential results, causing harm to those being surveyed).
- Inappropriate choice of sample, resulting in the wrong conclusions being drawn.
- Bias in the sample - e.g. there may have been a volunteer effect in which those who volunteered to take part in the study were found to provide different answers from non-volunteers.
- Respondent unreliability or reticence. Perhaps people did not tell the whole truth, refused to answer certain questions or gave dishonest but politically correct answers.
- Discovering after the survey had been sent out that a key question was omitted.
- Use of jargon or incomprehensible words in the survey design. Badly worded, ambiguous questions are very common in poorly thought out surveys.
- Poor relationship between the design of the question and the design of the scoring system, such as 'Would you prefer patient visits to start at 6 pm *or* 7 pm? when just a 'Yes'/'No' response format has been provided.
- Coding the data in an inappropriate manner (for example, grouping data into poorly thought out categories such as social class, marital status and ethnic background when none of these is relevant).
- Failure to use appropriate statistics to analyse the data.

Definition of terms

For convenience, the following terms are used within this book:

The Client: The person for whom the work is conducted and/or the people who review the quality of the survey after it is finished. The Client will not always be the initiator of a survey but this is the case in the vast majority of situations. Sometimes the Client will be a health manager and sometimes a team of people will be commissioning the work.

The Researcher: The person who conducts the work. The Researcher could be an internal person or external consultant and could conceivably also be the Client.

The Respondents: The people who complete the survey after it has been sent out. Respondents could be staff from all levels within and/or connected to the health organization, patients, the larger community from which patients are drawn, suppliers, etc.

How Clients and Researchers should use this book

Many readers will want to read the book in its entirety prior to embarking on their survey projects or commissioning a survey. However, if you wish to dip into various key sections then see the instant access chart below to read about the specific stages of the survey design process.

Major event	Action
Basic rationale	Purpose and general overview of surveys (p.3–71) ⇓
Client commissions a survey	Scientific approach to surveys (18) ⇓
	Survey objectives (20) and hypotheses (22) ⇓
	Ethics (27) ⇓

	Necessity of survey (32); Select, adapt or create a survey (33) ⇓
	Time to complete (44); Risks (45); Contract (45); Funding (49); Politics (49) ⇓
	Understand theory (54–61) and practice (61) ⇓
Survey begins to take shape	Plan the survey design (65–72) ⇓
	Choose between different types of survey - postal, interview, telephone, etc. (73–91) ⇓
Sampling requirements	Obtain representative sample (92–5) ⇓
Writing the survey items	Generate, choose and group the items (99–110) ⇓
	General format considerations (111–20) ⇓
	Choose type of item (120–31) ⇓
	Code the answer-sheet or think about using automatic data entry (131–2)
Evaluate the items	Qualitative method (137)
	For 'attitude' surveys also use a quantitative method (138–46). ⇓
Administer the survey	
Perform the data analysis	Select analysis method (156) ⇓
	Analyse the data (157–81)

Write and present the results	The report and presentation (185–90) ⇓
Client evaluation	Evaluate the quality of the work (191–7) ⇓
Example reports	Example reports with critiques (198)

Part 1
Background principles

Chapter 1
The basic rationale

Why do we need surveys and questionnaires?

All good management decisions are inevitably a function of the data upon which the decision is made. Before deciding how to increase staff morale, initiate a new treatment programme, improve patient satisfaction or assess local public opinion, decision makers need data about the present situation. They need to know who thinks what and why. They need to understand the nature of differences between various groups and how they see issues. Surveys and questionnaires have the potential to provide crucial evidence in this decision making process. The opposite side of the coin, however, is that surveys and questionnaires can be expensive and time-consuming. Before deciding to embark on the design of a questionnaire or survey, an organization needs to be able to justify the resources, time and effort required for successful completion of the survey.

The most obvious way in which surveys and questionnaires are used by health professionals is in the evaluation of patient care and patient treatment programmes. If a survey is conducted prior to the implementation of a care programme and then again after its completion, the effectiveness of the programme can be established. A before and after measure of success can be obtained by examining differences in the survey responses over these two time periods. Such evaluations may be objective (such as having a checklist of symptoms) or subjective by showing how major changes in attitudes and behaviours have occurred over time (such as asking about how well patients have coped with pain). With a growing interest in health psychology, there is an increasing interest in the measurement of psychological variables associated with health and illness. To minimize practice and prior knowledge effects, for example, quite often more elaborate designs are used in such studies. These designs involve the use of control groups (i.e. patients who are not receiving treatment), and 'blind' evaluation by clinicians who are unaware of whether the patient is in the programme or in a control group.

However, surveys and questionnaires are used within the health services for many other purposes than just patient evaluation. Health professionals work within large and complex organizations that need to collect information about themselves, their staff, their patients and how people experience and see their environment. Surveys are useful ways of collecting basic management information. Here is a list of some of the other uses of surveys and questionnaires within a health organization:

(a) To separate fact from opinion

A survey provides quantifiable information. Many doctors, administrators and others claim to know what patients and employees want, think and need. Often the only way to fight such ingrained opinion is to present factual survey information that goes beyond the 'gut feeling' beliefs of staff who may not always be in touch with patient or peer opinions. The quality of plans and objectives of the health service professional depends to a large extent on the quality of the information upon which these plans are made. All decisions and plans should require factual input, and this can include systematic feedback from survey respondents. Professionally conducted surveys can be expected to provide hard empirical data upon which solid, workable plans can be based.

(b) To obtain unbiased information

A report written from the evidence collected from a good survey or questionnaire will present facts rather than value judgements and show how preconceived notions on the part of many people are not necessarily objective truths. For example, it is common for management to see the way things are done through their own 'rose-coloured spectacles', ignoring or misinterpreting the ideas, beliefs and experiences of staff and patients. An attitude survey or questionnaire offers the Client the chance to collect information directly from appropriate people as opposed to relying on information that is filtered and changed as it passes though the different levels of the organization. A survey provides an upward flow of information towards management, whereas usually the flow of information is downwards from management.

(c) To know if the organization is meeting its objectives or is at risk

A survey or questionnaire can provide vital information to a client (such as the manager of a health organization) to determine if it is fulfilling its objectives as perceived by the customer (e.g. 90% patient satisfaction). This can be not only in terms of meeting planned targets but also whether or not the organization is meeting its legal and contractual obligations. This reduces the possibility of patient complaints, staff complaints and expensive lawsuits. Interestingly, whereas 'objective' criteria on certain factors may be collected (e.g. time delays) these criteria may not concur with patient or staff perceptions of them. Appropriate survey techniques can ultimately help organizations reach their targets.

(d) To identify opportunities for growth, change and improvement

A survey can be used to question a particular method, procedure or technique so that its effectiveness can be evaluated. A survey can therefore challenge the status quo in the light of changing circumstances. For example, surveys have been used to show a correlation between smoking and cancer. By conducting such surveys, it proved possible to begin the process of finding one of the main causes of cancer with the aim of improving life expectancy. Surveys have also identified staff dissatisfaction with appraisal systems, allowing them to be altered and improved to make them more equitable and understandable.

(e) To improve the morale and motivation of the respondents

A survey or questionnaire enables all the respondents (whether staff or patients) to express a viewpoint. This improvement in communication can improve morale and motivation at all levels directly as a result of balloting respondents for their opinions. Equally, of course, surveys can raise expectations, and if not acted upon, may lower morale and motivation. The idea that a survey is a vote of confidence or an upward feedback mechanism can work well to improve the morale of respondents, provided the results of the survey are acted on in a timely and open manner.

(f) To assess respondents' needs

A survey can produce a comprehensive assessment of staff training needs or patients' care needs. A survey can also provide an assessment of an individual's self-perceived effectiveness at his or her job. This type of survey can provide valuable extra information to the more traditional appraisal process. This is especially valuable in cases where managers dislike the feeling that they are sitting in judgement or have concerns that personal feelings may cloud the issue and render their judgements less than accurate.

(g) To assess the status and capability of equipment and buildings, etc.

A survey can be used to assess the status and capability of equipment or buildings within the organization by assessing physical condition, maintenance requirements, repair and fault history, as well as the need for modified equipment to perform new procedures. A survey can also help to show the effectiveness of preventative maintenance or condition monitoring systems and assess whether or not, in the light of technological advances and competitors' activities, the equipment wastes resources (such as floor space or energy). A survey can also determine users' attitudes towards equipment and buildings, whether state-of-the-art or old-fashioned. Changing old-fashioned, less reliable and less efficient equipment is frequently, and perhaps surprisingly to some, not accepted as being self-evidently beneficial.

(h) To provide insight into recruitment and selection

By selecting (or rejecting) people with specific preferences, values and potentialities, it is possible to both maintain and to change a corporate culture. Some organizations are very careful to select employees from a particular background knowing that they share common beliefs, attitudes and values. Surveys can be used in 'exit interviews' or to assess the selection experience of those accepted and rejected by the organization. Some questionnaires, on the other hand, are used in the selection process itself, for example, to measure personality, values or expectations.

(i) To measure the culture of the organization

Surveys of staff show the homogeneity or heterogeneity of a department or organization as a whole so that action plans may be developed. For example, based on a culture survey, the client may wish to change corporate culture and identity by recruiting a more heterogeneous group who do not share the same beliefs and values. Culture or climate questionnaires can be very useful as an index of 'before' and 'after' radical change within an organization. They can also be used to explain patterns of friction within an organization and why certain groups respond to change in the way they do.

(j) To provide insight into patients' backgrounds
Health organizations draw their patients from different cultural, class and geographical locations. Surveys of patients' backgrounds provide information to the health professional so that resources can be more accurately allocated to where they are needed most. For example, in a predominantly Arabic-speaking part of London, England, it may be necessary to have Arabic signs, Arabic interpreters and Arabic food on the menu.

(k) To assist in the assessment of staff training
It is often very difficult to determine whether training courses are worthwhile investments. A survey or questionnaire can provide useful information about training for the personnel who participate. These surveys yield information about who has been trained on what, their reactions to courses and any perceived further training needs. One can also take a look at attitudes, beliefs and knowledge before and after a course, as well as some time later when they can be related to actual changes in workplace practice.

(l) To show potential fit and misfit in mergers, acquisitions and partnerships
In the search for the best-value treatment of patients, many health organizations throughout the world are being subjected to increasing scrutiny and change. Surveys are used to guide policy and strategic development. Surveys are also used to determine the level of difficulty two hospitals, departments, trusts, etc., would have if they were to merge. By surveying aspects of two organizations before the merger, it is possible to determine the nature, extent and implications of a merger between them.

(m) To show the quality of work and staff during 'quality audits'
Public and private health organizations are increasingly accountable to commissions, inspectorates and other bodies for their behaviour and the quality of their work. Surveys can be used to present direct and unbiased evidence of the quality of work and quality of staff. For example, student feedback from nurse training

is regarded as very important for judging whether or not students are satisfied with their courses from a particular institution.

A brief overview of the survey process

When conducting a survey, it is very important for the Researcher to have an overall plan of action. Each of these points will be explored in greater detail in later sections:

(a) Formulate the objectives explicitly but examine them from all perspectives
Prior to designing and implementing a questionnaire or survey, there is an important preliminary stage of development. In this stage, the Researcher consults with the Client to determine the objectives of the project and secures the commitment of the Client to see all steps of the survey through to completion. The Researcher should secure a clear, explicit, *written contract* covering all the phases of the project. The Client will need to be briefed on how the project will progress with the Researcher constantly underlining the necessity for the Client to take an active role to ensure the success of the survey and the need to act upon the survey's results. Ethical and financial considerations need to be planned and the Researcher needs to know that the Clients will give enough time to the project before they want to see the results.

Once the survey objectives have been formulated, the Researcher will need to do some research to understand the nature of the problem and to determine if a survey is necessary. Perhaps the questions have already been asked in a survey that has already been published? Perhaps the information could be obtained better using some other method? Given that the survey technique has been decided upon, the Researcher may wish to use a known, published, off-the-shelf, survey; adapt a survey that has been used in the past; or start from scratch and create one. Clearly, there are many cost and time advantages to using a survey that has already been designed, but the Researcher needs to be sure that such surveys will meet the Client's objectives.

(b) Design the survey instrument
Given that the Researcher decides to design a questionnaire from scratch, the next step is to plan the general shape of the survey.

Another important question to consider at this time is the administration method. The most general choice here is between a 'postal' or an interview method. After this the items in the survey can be formulated and written.

(c) Test (or pilot) the survey
Next the survey is tested among a small representative pilot sample of Respondents to check applicability, misunderstandings and ambiguities concerning the instructions and the questions. This stage is completed by finalizing the survey contents and gaining the final agreement of the Client. The success of the survey will depend upon the survey questionnaire being comprehensive, user-friendly, succinct, unambiguous and relevant.

(d) Administer (or run) the questionnaire
At long last the survey is administered to the Respondents (e.g. by hand, post, telephone, structured interview, in groups, etc.). The appropriate sampling method will have been used to ensure the data are representative. It is important to be sure of the sample because, without proper understanding of the principles involved in obtaining a representative sample, conclusions drawn will be of doubtful validity.

If the questionnaires are posted to the Respondents, then a time limit will need to be decided upon and the expected date of return clearly indicated. Late returns will need to be chased up to ensure as large a response rate as possible. The questionnaires need to be collated and then returned to the Researcher for analysis.

(e) Analysis, presentation and beyond
The final stage is to analyse the data, preferably by computer. Results are usually statistically analysed at first in terms of percentage of Respondents who indicate agreement or disagreement (or whatever other classification has been used) to various items. Often the mean scores are also used. Items subsumed under a particular heading may also be reported as total or average scores for the category as a whole. Results are often presented as tables, graphs or charts. If the Researcher has the expertise, then much more about the Respondents can often be learned by the use of multivariate statistical methods (such as factor analysis

and multiple regression). These advanced techniques can summarize the different categories of perceptions from different Respondents and reveal predictive models that will guide programmes in the future. For example, it may be possible to determine which demographic factors (age, sex, class, ethnicity) predict a particular aspect of nursing care.

The end result of the survey is a report and presentation of the results to the Client. In general, however, the process does not stop here. Action plans will need to be drawn up and targets set so that the issues raised by the survey are addressed. There may be a need to perform a survey again at a later stage to determine if the targets that were set have been reached. Repeat surveys can be useful to plot trends over time, thereby allowing the Client to determine if changes are occurring and whether the rate of change is acceptable.

What is best practice?

Whatever the motives of the people commissioning the survey, and whether or not they follow good practice in their decision making, the Researcher who conducts a survey should *always* follow best practice guidelines. Best practice is about doing the survey right and therefore providing the survey sponsors with accurate and reliable information upon which their future decision making will be based. Of course, 'best practice' is something of a subjective perception and different groups of people have different ideas of what is, and what is not, best practice. By 'best practice' we mean following the correct, state-of-the-art procedures that are benchmarked by both academic and practical criteria.

Researchers should follow best practice for the following reasons:

(a) Best practice provides quality results and the most accurate information for the Client. Anything other than best practice may mean that the Researcher is providing results of dubious merit.
(b) Best practice is what Clients expect *even when they say otherwise*. Anything other than best practice will always mean that the Client is eventually unhappy with the work. Whatever Clients say during a project, they will always say that best practice is what they were expecting, especially when things go wrong. For example, a Client may encourage corner-cutting at the early stage of a

project to keep costs low, and yet still blame the Researcher for poor management of the project when it turns out to have been fatally flawed by these cuts.
(c) Best practice means that the Researcher is protected if things should go wrong.
(d) Unless best practice is followed, things inevitably will go wrong!
(e) Researchers who follow best practice guidelines will in general be happier and more satisfied with their life at work than those who do not.

Best practice in conducting a survey involves selecting and using the optimal methods at all times, whether in the planning, design, administration, scoring or interpretation of the results. In the course of this book it will become clear that although all these stages are crucial, the earlier ones are arguably the most important. If errors are made here, then the rest must inevitably be wrong as well. For example, the whole project may be fatally undermined if a meaningless or ambiguous question is mistakenly included in a questionnaire and not spotted until the end of the analysis. On the other hand, a mistake in the statistical analysis might also undermine the project if it is not spotted, but once spotted it can be rectified.

Best practice is not just about getting it right; it is also about what to do when things have gone wrong. First and foremost, it is essential that a Researcher acknowledges mistakes when they are made (and they will be!) and admits to them, as opposed to covering them up and hoping they will go away. It is only by being open in one's work that it is possible to develop a professional reputation for competence and to learn from negative experiences so that things go right in the future. Best practice is therefore more than just a series of rules about how to conduct an optimal survey; indeed it is a philosophical approach to work, advocating a strategy that will make both you and the organization successful.

General characteristics of a good survey

During the planning stages it is essential to keep an overview of the survey design in mind, because minor points that are overlooked can turn out to have major significance at a later stage. A good survey design will take into account the process of administering the survey and the finished product. With surveys, the end result depends on the effort that is put into understanding the real purpose of the project, as well as getting all the minor details right. The major characteristics of a good survey are:

(a) It measures the right things, and can distinguish the wood from the trees
An effective survey depends upon having a clear idea about aims and objectives. What is the survey going to measure? Preliminary stages of a survey design need to concentrate on establishing the main goals of the survey; in short, what exactly has to be surveyed and why.

(b) It has clear, well thought-through dimensions or categories of what to measure.
It is very important to be sure about the dimensions and categories that are to be measured. For instance, imagine you are measuring phobias. Phobias seem to fall into three categories: inanimate objects (needles, scissors), animate objects (snakes, birds, mice) and ambiguous situations (the dark, heights). To get a good measure of phobias *all* the above categories need to be sampled. It may also be important to measure the level of importance of these dimensions, and the degree of overlap between the dimensions may need to be ascertained. For example, the fear of crowds might be classified as an ambiguous or an animate phobia depending upon perspective. Usually it is difficult to put all the relevant items into categories within a survey. When this happens the Researcher will have to recognize that the categories are not perfect.

(c) It is user-friendly
Some surveys and questionnaires are written in impenetrable management jargon or psychobabble. It takes skill and time to devise clear, unambiguous, logically constructed questions that tap into the relevant dimensions and do not use acronyms or emotionally loaded words. Surveys need to be simple to complete in order to provide useful and valid data. This is especially true if the survey is aimed at a broad section of the general public.

(d) It is simple and brief
Surveys need to be succinct but comprehensive. It is not unreasonable to ask 100 questions, and such a survey can take less than half an hour to complete. It is therefore important that only the most pertinent 100 questions are asked. Length, quality and overall usefulness are not related to each other. Wise Researchers are

parsimonious and ask as few questions as possible, although they will be the most differentiating questions.
(e) It is tailored to the Client's needs
Every survey needs to be tailored towards the needs of the organization for which it is intended. All organizations have their own specific meanings for words and their own unique concepts that need to be considered. Does the Researcher know what kind of report is required? How much detail should it contain? Who is going to receive it? What kind of statistics will the Client understand?

Answering unfounded criticism

For some in the health professions, the business of psychological auditing by means of a survey or questionnaire is mysterious, threatening and perhaps even regarded as dangerous. Some health professionals and administrators often resist any form of data collection by putting forward various spurious, easily refuted arguments. Although informed criticism is vital to ensuring best practice and should therefore be encouraged, those interested in surveys and questionnaires need to be aware of the likely unfounded criticism so that they are adequately prepared with counter-arguments:

(a) You cannot measure abstract things such as staff or patient attitudes
A favourite argument against conducting a survey is that surveys cannot be relied upon to provide an accurate and sensitive measure of abstract organizational attributes such as attitudes, climate, culture or morale. However, when properly designed using best practice guidelines, surveys can effectively tap into the attitudes, beliefs, intentions and opinions of various groups. In short, well-designed surveys have been shown to be valid because their results generally seem able to predict useful behaviours.
(b) You cannot tell what particular information to collect
Whenever a survey is conducted, it is important for the Researcher to carry out preparatory exercises to define the nature of the problems or questions that need to be measured. Many useful clues as to what the survey or questionnaire should address can be obtained through pilot work (initial interviews with key individuals, open-ended discussions with small groups of staff or

patients or both, and so on). To a large extent the purpose of a survey tends to make it very clear what kinds of information need to be collected. Pilot studies and focus groups will usually be sufficient to determine what information to collect.

(c) You cannot determine the return on the investment and so it does not make accounting sense to conduct a survey

It is true that a survey's 'value for money' can rarely be demonstrated. However the cost of *not* doing a survey is easily demonstrated. Poor treatments, failed mergers, inadequately trained staff, dissatisfied patients and low morale are just some of the problems that can result from not knowing about what happens within a health organization. An early survey may identify the problems and indicate ways of avoiding them before management mistakes are made.

(d) You can provide senior management with a report but they will not read it

It is true that senior management are often over-burdened with paperwork but if the results of the survey are important (do not bother doing any other kind!) then the relevant managers will not ignore the results. Indeed an executive summary with some counter-intuitive or myth-breaking findings will usually guarantee that senior management reads the report from cover to cover. In fact, unless the organization has been chronically over-surveyed, then most managers avidly read the reports, especially the sections about themselves. In fact, they can be so interested that they go to great lengths to keep them secret!

(e) You cannot measure all the relevant details in a survey

A good survey can take into account all the identified factors that are relevant and salient. That is, one can measure attitudes, beliefs, past behaviours and values that are associated with a particular event. Most surveys are multidimensional and the use of multivariate statistical techniques can measure individual or combined effects of any of the major variables that influence survey responses. Clearly, however, such types of survey methods are much more involved and require a degree of experience that many survey 'first-timers' will be ill-equipped to undertake.

(f) You can exacerbate staff and patient discontent with a survey

If done properly, surveys can reduce rather than worsen organizational problems because they actually provide a much sought after mechanism to let management know what staff and patients think. Indeed, people can safely let off steam with a survey. Otherwise they might express their dissatisfaction and discontent in more serious and destructive ways (e.g. absenteeism, tribunals, official complaints, resignation). Problems with surveys can occur, however, when results are not acted upon or are kept secret by an inward-looking management team who believe that bad news (and inevitably there will be some) means that the report should be suppressed.

(g) You cannot trust the results of a survey
Management are not always convinced by the honesty and accuracy of a technique that invites personal views. Staff and patients also may distrust the motives of management for carrying out a survey and will need to be convinced that the survey is worthwhile and will improve their situation. Scepticism can easily be overcome if a survey is done in a detailed and professional manner. If done by an outside Researcher who has nothing to gain politically, then employee scepticism against a particularly sensitive type of survey can be much alleviated. Equally, anonymity and confidentiality are important issues with regard to achieving the trust of the people completing the questionnaire.

What formal qualifications do I need to undertake research?

Your interest in designing a survey with a view to best practice is the best qualification of all. Whether you are the Client or the Researcher, formal qualifications may be of help in the design of a survey or questionnaire. However, experience and practice is probably an even better qualification. Our experience is that people who are well qualified on paper can often seriously underestimate the complexities of survey and questionnaire design. First-timers and novices would do well to find the services of a mentor to oversee their work and to be available for discussion of the more complex issues.

Internal versus external Researcher?

Organizations will inevitably have to consider the value, or otherwise, of employing their own permanent member of staff whose duties consist solely of conducting surveys. The decision depends upon a number of factors, including the size of the organization and the importance attached to information gathering. Large organizations can generally justify and sustain the cost of in-house Researchers who have the advantage of in-depth inside information about how the organization works. The internal Researcher (e.g. a line manager or internal consultant) therefore has the advantage of knowing the organization and being in tune with existing ways of doing things. On the other hand, the external Researcher has the advantage of independence and confidentiality; staff and patients may feel more relaxed and able to divulge opinions on sensitive issues.

Edwards, Thomas, Rosenfeld and Booth-Kewley (1997) suggest that the use of non-specialist internal Researchers can be a poor choice in terms of efficient utilization of resources. For example, highly paid internal Researchers may end up stuffing and opening the envelopes in which the surveys are sent, and entering the data themselves. They suggest that, at the very least, it is much better to employ external contractors to do these chores even if the internal Researchers do the more intellectual activities involved in the survey process. A summary of the advantages and disadvantages of the two types of Researcher is shown in Table 1.

Table 1. Advantages and disadvantages of using internal versus external Researchers

Internal consultant	External consultant
Maintains confidentiality within the organization	Might divulge information to competitors
Greater immediate understanding of the problem	Need time to understand problem
Know how to get the project going	Need internal contacts to get the job done
May not be efficient	Usually efficient
May not be experienced	Usually experienced
May not have the right equipment	Usually well equipped
May not be trusted by management	Usually trusted by management
May not be able to ensure confidentiality	Can usually assure confidentiality to subjects
Seems cheap but may be expensive	Seems expensive but may be 'cheaper'

Please note that these comparisons are, of course, generalizations since all organizations and external agencies are different.

Summary

Surveys and questionnaires are used throughout the health professions in a variety of ways. Their applicability is wide and their usefulness in providing information is great. Wise Researchers will use best practice in their design and the Client should always keep these principles in mind when commissioning or evaluating the results of a survey or questionnaire. Without following best practice guidelines, it is almost inevitable that mistakes will be made. Researchers should also be sure that they are suitably qualified and prepared to undertake survey work and that they can answer the relatively standard ill-informed criticism of survey work that will generally be thrown at them by critical colleagues. Clients need to choose between internal and external Researchers.

Chapter 2
Determining objectives and hypotheses

Introduction

A management team usually has a vague idea that some information needs to be collected so that better decisions can be made. A member of the team approaches a Researcher and asks if this research can be undertaken to help the management make the decisions. This is the typical scenario which sets off a chain of actions that can result in a survey being commissioned. The first step of the Researcher is to work with the client to formulate correctly the objectives and the hypotheses of the study.

Using the scientific approach

To follow best practice in survey design, it is always necessary to follow the general principles of what is known as the *scientific method* (see Figure 1). To use scientific principles properly, the following steps need to be followed:

(a) The Researcher needs to be aware that a problem or an area of research exists that needs an explanation or at least a better description. The problem needs careful definition, and this provides the objective or purpose of the survey. Clearly, without a purpose a survey has no usefulness. What precisely do the clients want to know? How do they want the results presented? Do they have a model that they want tested? Do they have several hypotheses about something that they would like investigated?

Determining objectives and hypotheses

(b) Find out as much about the research topic as possible. It is necessary to understand the problem in order to design the survey, and this usually takes the form of research in the library followed by an analysis of the practical nature of the research topic.

(c) Come up with a first guess as to the answer to the problem. This is the first hypothesis *(e.g. men tend to visit the doctor less than women because they have less faith in doctors)*, but bear in mind that more than one hypothesis can be tested at any one time.

It may be that the purpose of the survey or questionnaire is purely to gather information, and, if this is true, then it may not be strictly necessary to generate hypotheses. Nevertheless the Clients are almost always interested in testing one or more hypotheses. *For example, the Clients of a project say they would like information about the length of time consultants spend travelling to work. It is, in fact, much better to go back to the Clients and ask them precisely why they want this information. They might say it is because they are concerned that consultants live too far away to be able to respond to emergencies. The hypothesis to test is therefore that 'consultants live too far away to be able to respond to emergencies'.* As can be seen, hypotheses are the key to understanding and defining the problem in a scientific manner. Without the hypothesis the survey loses its direction, may not answer the research question and may identify only superficial aspects of the research problem.

(d) A survey or questionnaire (if either is the best method) needs to be developed to investigate the problem in as objective a manner as possible. This may involve asking various questions to determine if any particular set of questions provides the most logical explanation of the phenomenon to be investigated. More complex designs may involve performing an experiment in which conditions are manipulated in order to determine whether they get the expected reaction. *For example, the Client is interested in determining whether a particular training course will reduce race and gender effects on the quality of treatment provided. Here there may be 'before' and 'after' conditions in which racial and gender effects are investigated.*

(e) The data generated from the survey are analysed to determine if there is any evidence in favour of the hypothesis. The hypothesis may have to be revised, and if this is the case, then further investigation of the problem must be undertaken in order to prove this new hypothesis. If the first hypothesis is correct, then it will probably need to be refined and further investigated, possibly using another survey or some other technique such as in-depth interviewing.

(f) If the predictions made were correct, then the proposed explanation was probably correct. Otherwise, it is necessary to start again and derive further hypotheses to be tested.

Define objective(s)

⇓

Review literature, observe and understand the problem

⇓

Formulate hypotheses that explain the research issue

⇓

Design survey to test the hypotheses

⇓

Carry out survey

⇓

Analyse results

⇓

Do results support the hypothesis? If not then develop an alternative and conduct a further study

---

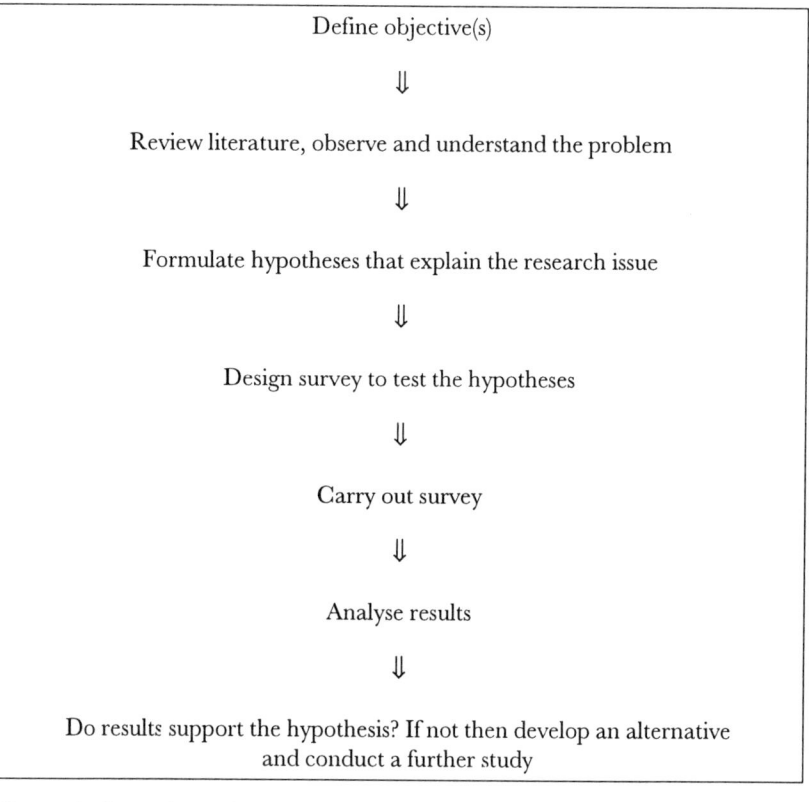

Figure 1. Overview of the scientific approach to survey design

Understanding the Client's objective

The first thing the Researcher must do is to determine the Client's objective in collecting the survey information. Often the Client will not have a clear idea (it may be ambiguous, unrealistic or just flawed!), and so further discussion will be required. It is only when the Researcher is clear about the real objective of the survey that it can be written down in a clear and precise manner. *For example, the Client is worried about low morale amongst junior doctors. Can the Researcher*

Determining objectives and hypotheses 21

identify the source of it? Here 'morale' could have a multitude of meanings (e.g. job dissatisfaction, high turnover, large amount of absenteeism or sickness, poor work conditions, poor pay, large number of hours worked, poor accommodation). In this situation, the Researcher needs to discover whether the Client really wants a general survey or something more precise and directed.

It is crucial to get the research objective right from the start. The following objectives are quite vague:

(a) Doctor–patient interaction
(b) Dentistry in inner cities
(c) Problems with hospital visitors
(d) Nursing practice
(e) Administration of midwives

whereas the following objectives can be regarded as much less vague:

(a) Patients' attitudes towards quality of food
(b) Women's beliefs about home births
(c) Differences in job satisfaction amongst management and staff
(d) Attitudes towards HIV patients in the community
(e) Allocation of pay bonuses to cleaning staff
(f) Degree to which instructions on drug administration are followed.

Couchman and Dawson (1990) provide examples of vague and clear words which may be of help to the Researcher in stating the objectives of the survey:

Vague	**Clear**
knowing	comparing
understanding	contrasting
appreciating	constructing
developing	defining
internalizing	discriminating
enjoying	sorting

The way in which a broad research question can be narrowed down to a specific research question can be illustrated with the following example. *The Clients come to the Researcher and say they are* worried about the long hours worked by junior doctors. This would be a vague, ambiguous and broad objective. The Researcher then determines the specific worries of the Clients. These turn out to be related to the types of mistakes in medical practice that can result from too many hours on duty. A formal research statement would then be translated into: 'Common errors of decision making made by junior doctors as a result of fatigue'. Notice that the objective is quite different from the original problem voiced by the Clients.

It is also easy for the Client and the Researcher to confuse completely the nature of the project and great care should be taken by the Researcher to ensure that the Client's true aims are identified. For example, the Client claims to want a survey about the extent to which staff follow guidelines for the administration of dangerous drugs. A Researcher should want to know why the Client is interested in this particular issue. Is it because the Client is worried about stress effects on staff, worried that the guidelines are not being adhered to, worried that drugs are going missing or some other thing? Each of these different perspectives would lead to a very different type of survey with very different objectives and hypotheses to test.

The objective checklist

(a) Is the objective clearly defined?
(b) Can it be written down unambiguously and succinctly?
(c) Try to cover the what, where, when and how as well as outcome of the proposed research.
(d) Has the Researcher taken one last look at the objective and made sure that anyone could read it and gain a good idea of what is intended?
(e) Has the Researcher checked as to whether the Clients are happy with the way the objective has been stated?
(f) Is the Client aware that the scope of the project will depend largely upon the breadth of the objective?

Deriving hypotheses from the objective

If the objective of the survey project is clear, then it will be much easier to draw hypotheses. A hypothesis is a prediction concerning what the findings will be, i.e. how variables relate to each other (such as male and female doctors' reactions to stress). It is this prediction, as opposed to the objective, that is tested by means of a survey or questionnaire. Following the statement of the objective, the

Researcher will usually formulate one or more hypotheses for empirical testing. Whereas the objective is typically a phrase describing the project or a question about a problem, the hypotheses are tentative predictions of the findings that are specific and testable. Hypotheses are usually formulated before data collection because the hypotheses provide the direction for the project, promote critical thinking and tell us which results will provide positive support for what is being tested and which will provide negative support. Because in survey or questionnaire research it is almost always possible to explain results in a variety of different ways, hypotheses written before data collection serve to guard against data being misconstrued. Except for the most simple descriptive type of survey or questionnaire, there is simply no way that a Researcher can avoid the need for hypotheses, and so it is essential that the Researcher understands what they are right from the start.

A hypothesis states a relationship between more than one variable. Thus a simple type of hypothesis will state a relationship between a single independent variable (X) and a dependent variable (Y). The dependent variable is the predicted effect or outcome of manipulating the independent variable, which is presumed to be a cause or antecedent of the dependent variable. A complex type of hypothesis is likely to contain more than one independent variable (X1, X2, X3) as predictors of the dependent variable (Y) or several dependent variables (Y1, Y2, Y3). Complex hypotheses are useful because they mirror problems found in the real world, but they add to the complexity of the study and are more difficult to test.

A few examples are given here, but see Polit and Hungler (1991) for a selection of good examples from the nursing profession:

Example 1
Objective
To determine whether the presence of the father makes the birth process more satisfying for the mother

Hypothesis
Presence of the father in childbirth causes the birth experience of the mother to be more satisfying

Independent variable
X Presence of father

Dependent variable
Y Birth satisfaction questionnaire completed by the mother after giving birth

---

Example 2
Objective
To identify some predictors of life expectancy

Research problem
Patient sense of health and good diet predict life expectancy

Independent variables
X1 Sense of health questionnaire
X2 Diet questionnaire

Dependent variable
Y Age of death

Example 3
Objective
To determine whether alcohol consumption by patients has beneficial effects

Hypothesis
Intake of alcohol is related to better health and morale of patients

Independent variable
X Number of units of alcohol consumed

Dependent variables
Y1 Sense of health questionnaire
Y2 Morale questionnaire

Example 4
Objective
To determine whether dentists are satisfied with their pay and conditions

Hypothesis
The majority of dentists are satisfied with their pay and conditions

Independent variable
X Proportion of dentists expressing satisfaction from a survey

Dependent variables
Y1 Amount of pay received
Y2 Questionnaire about different factors associated with work conditions

(therefore probably specifying Y2 in terms of these work conditions)

Hypotheses are never proven or disproven by means of a survey, questionnaire or even by more formal experimentation. All a study can do is add evidence in support of a hypothesis or provide evidence against a hypothesis. A classic example illustrates this point. An experimenter has a hypothesis that 'all swans are white'. This dynamic person sets out to collect an extremely large and representative sample of the population of swans, and sure enough comes up with a conclusion that all swans sampled in the survey are white. This does not prove the issue, however; it 'merely' adds strong evidence in favour of the hypothesis.

Our final point is that there are two types of hypothesis. The first is the research hypothesis, i.e. what the Researchers expect to find in their research. All the above examples are research hypotheses. This is the way that most hypotheses are expressed. However, from the statistical perspective it needs to be noted that the hypotheses to be tested are *null hypotheses* in which *no* relationship between the independent and dependent variables is stated. In other words, statistical tests determine whether or not there is evidence in favour of rejecting a null hypothesis. Thus, in Example 1 above the null hypothesis is that there is *no* relationship between the mother's satisfaction and the presence of the father. The Researcher would then determine whether the correlation between these variables was significantly different from zero (in other words the null hypothesis would be tested). If the correlation was significant, the Researcher would then conclude that the null hypothesis could be rejected (thus providing evidence in favour of the research hypothesis).

All this will sound a bit complex and confusing to the novice Researcher but the concept of statistical testing is extremely important and needs to be understood. To summarize:

(a) most hypotheses are phrased to suggest that a relationship exists between two or more variables;
(b) the null hypothesis (that there is no relationship between the variables) is what is tested.

If the test is shown to be significant, then the null hypothesis is rejected and support is therefore offered for the research hypothesis; if the test is not significant, then the null hypothesis is accepted and no relationship between the variables is found.

Summary

Once a client approaches the Researcher with the research plan, it is generally up to the Researcher to reformulate the original idea so that the objectives are clear and hypotheses can be derived.

Chapter 3
Under what circumstances should the survey be undertaken?

Introduction

Once the Researcher has had a chance to clarify the objectives and derive hypotheses, it is possible to determine whether a survey really needs to be undertaken at all. There may be all sorts of reasons why the survey may need to be reformulated, or why the project may not need to be undertaken at all.

The ethics

Of prime importance to the Researcher and the Client, who commissions the work, is the ethical dimension to a survey or questionnaire project. Ethics refer to rules of conduct and whether or not the work conforms to existing guidelines as supplied by government bodies, professional associations or local committees. For example, the British Psychological Society (BPS) and the American Psychological Association (APA) provide codes of conduct which list rules for members. Failure to follow such rules could lead to a member of the society or association being disciplined or even struck off.

Polit and Hungler (1991) summarize the three fundamental ethical principles upon which ethical standards of behaviour can be based:

(a) The principle of beneficence
 The basic rule here is to do no form of harm to the Respondents. The Researcher should carefully evaluate the cost:benefit ratio on behalf of the Respondents and must weigh the risks to the subjects against the benefits to society.

(b) The principle of human dignity
   This principle includes the subjects' right to self-determination, which means that the Respondents should have the freedom to control their own activity, including the right not to take part in the study. Respondents should normally also have full knowledge about the experiment (the right to full disclosure). When the Researcher does not provide full disclosure, such as when it is felt that this will bias the results, then the Researcher might engage in covert data collection, concealment or deception. There is debate about the ethics of such methods and the Researcher should take extra care in these situations to ensure the rights of, and minimize the risks to, the subjects. Some ethics committees are likely to take a dim view of any infringements of the right to full disclosure.

(c) The principle of justice
   Here Respondents have the right to fair treatment and privacy. Privacy can be achieved through anonymity and by ensuring that the procedures used are confidential. A Researcher should certainly also take into account the degree of inconvenience to Respondents and their likely emotional involvement. If there is a possibility of even a small breach in ethical rules then it is common to present all Respondents with a consent form that they must sign prior to answering the survey questions. *For example, a Researcher is interested in determining the types of contraception used by married women. The intrusive nature of the research dictates that the Respondents are asked to sign a consent form. If the Respondents had been young teenagers then it would also be wise to obtain parental consent.* In fact, consent forms can also give rise to ethical dilemmas so even these should be used with care. There have been cases in recent times when courts have attempted to seize such forms with a view to identifying the individuals concerned. In such a situation, it may be best to proceed informally and not use a consent form. However, the support and advice of an ethics committee would also usually be necessary in such situations.

In many settings within the health professions, there is a requirement that all research work (including surveys) is vetted by an ethics committee. This should consist of an informed but impartial group of individuals whose duty is to ensure that, among other things, the benefits of the study are greater than the cost, and that the cost (not just financial but also including physiological and psychological health, time spent, etc.) of the survey to the Respondents is not too great. Sometimes it may be necessary for a Researcher or an ethics committee to obtain legal advice or the advice of more experienced researchers in the field. This is required particularly when the Respondents are vulnerable - such as children, the elderly, the disabled or people with learning difficulties - or when very sensitive questions are asked.

Once the objective is clearly defined, the Researcher should consider the possible consequences of the survey. Even with the best of intentions, Clients may be planning a survey with objectives that are inappropriate or unethical. If this is the case, this is the time for the Researcher to object. Clearly such a situation requires sensitivity, but the Researcher may need to seek changes to the objectives or even refuse to undertake the project. The Researcher may be loath to do this, but unless action is taken at the beginning of the project, the consequences can only build up as time goes on.

For example, the Clients ask a Researcher to design a survey to provide evidence that domestic staff are satisfied with their pay. Here the issue is that the Clients have specified an inappropriate objective. The Researcher must return to the Clients and propose that the objective be rephrased to measure the satisfaction with pay in an unbiased manner so that the outcome is not specified before the study is conducted. It may also be that the Clients are interested in showing that domestic staff are satisfied with their pay for unethical reasons. Researchers should tread carefully in these situations and should remember that an unbiased and clearly stated objective is often a good way of identifying the ethics of the study.

The Researcher may also wish to inform the Client that surveys can be very damaging if there is no intention to correct problems that are identified. There is only one thing worse than doing nothing about a major source of dissatisfaction amongst staff. This is raising it as an issue and thus creating the expectation that something will be done about it, and then doing nothing. *For example, a hospital is interested in determining why it is difficult to retain the services of midwives. The hospital administrators widely advertise the fact that the matter is being attended to. The first step, they say, is to administer a survey and the second step is to take action on the results of the survey. That way resources can be channelled to where they are most required. The survey goes ahead but the results are not liked by the hospital (for example, a major conclusion is that management is poor). The hospital managers decide to keep the results of the survey confidential and decide not to progress further. There is no step two. If all this happens, and it does only too often, then the survey will end up having a negative effect on staff because their expectations were raised and then dashed. It would have been better if no survey had been conducted.*

Sometimes the Client and Researchers find themselves in an ethical dilemma (see Box 1). For example, they might be worried that informed consent will bias the results of the study. Although this may sometimes be the case, it can also be true that the danger of bias is overestimated. For example, Wiles (1988) advises that patients and nursing staff should be told what to expect before ward nurses are evaluated on their ability to provide good patient care. Although it could be expected that this prior information would alter the behaviour of the nurses, Wiles reports that the nurses seem to forget the presence of their evaluators and quickly become used to being observed. In this case the job of the evaluator is to observe and not intervene. However, Wiles adds that the only time the observers can intervene is when they ethically must - i.e. when they believe that the patient or the nurse is at risk.

The literature on health research (e.g. Polit & Hungler, 1991) provides some examples of modern studies that are unethical. The medical experiments conducted during the 1930s and 1940s in Nazi Germany are perhaps the most infamous of all. These experiments were unethical because they subjected the human subjects to physical harm and death, and because the subjects were not provided with the opportunity to refuse participation. The Tuskegee Syphilis Study (between 1932 and 1972) is a further example of an unethical study. The study, sponsored by the US Public Health Service, involved the deliberate withholding of treatment from men in a poor black community to determine the effects of syphilis when untreated. A third well-known case involved the injection of live cancer cells into elderly patients, without the consent of the patients, in the Jewish Chronic Disease Hospital in Brooklyn. These studies are just a few of the most famous cases which underline the need to give ethics a high profile when conducting research. Examples of ethical dilemmas to do with surveys are shown in Box 1.

In summary, therefore, an understanding of the ethical dimension to survey design leads to several possible conclusions:

(a) The survey is unethical and there is no alternative way of collecting the information. *For example, researchers have an interest in surveying the health of people who have been prescribed a certain pharmaceutical drug which is banned. Since the drug is banned, it would be exceedingly difficult to* run this survey without engaging in illegal and consequently unethical behaviour. It should be noted, however, that the law does not always have much to say about ethics. For example, a Researcher is interested in laboratory technicians' attitudes to animals undergoing non-legal surgery to investigate the effect of a drug. Such a survey may well be legal, but a Researcher may view it as unavoidably unethical.

Box 1

Some ethical dilemmas of surveys in the health professions

(a) How sensitive are doctors in their treatment of patients at health centres?
Ethical problem: It is generally extremely important from an ethical point of view to inform subjects of the nature of the research. Yet if the doctors are told that their empathy towards patients is being evaluated then it seems as though the purpose of the study will be undermined because the doctors may improve their sensitivity during the study, only to revert to their 'true' levels once the observers have departed.

(b) What are the feelings of parents after they have been told that their child has a serious illness?
Ethical problem: A study of this kind will intrude into the life of parents at a time when they are very vulnerable. This kind of probing can be both painful and traumatic.

(c) A survey to identify work absenteeism of senior hospital doctors with a view to their dismissal, when the survey states that the information will be used to improve work conditions.
Ethical problem: Such a survey would be designed to deceive the respondents and gain their participation through this deception.

All these dilemmas are not really dilemmas at all since the ethical issue cannot be 'got around'. In situations (a) and (c) there must be full disclosure of the nature of the project for the survey to proceed. If this is not satisfactory to the Client then the project must be looked at again. Situation (b) suggests that very careful thought must be put into the project to ensure that it is ethical and that the Respondents' needs are properly addressed.

(b) The survey design is unethical but an alternative and ethical way of conducting it is identified. *For example, a Researcher is interested in determining how nurses respond to dissatisfied patients. It would not be ethical to select patients at random and treat them so badly that they became dissatisfied simply to monitor the effect on nurses' morale. A better survey would be conducted by following up the situations when it became known that a patient was dissatisfied. The consequence of the change in survey design is that the Researcher loses control of the sample of patients and thus limits some of the conclusions that can be made from the study.*

(c) The research is ethical from the outset. *For example, the survey is aimed at collecting information about job satisfaction with a view to improving staff working conditions.*

Is the survey really necessary?

It may be that the information the Client needs already exists and therefore the Client's requirements are easily met with just a little research. It is also true to say that so many surveys are conducted in the health professions that yet another one may just involve a repeat of a previous one that has already been carefully constructed and administered. Given this need to regulate the number of surveys that members of the health professions must complete, the Researcher should:

(a) consider if the Client's questions can be added to a survey already in existence or if the research question has already been satisfactorily answered.

(b) evaluate whether the Client's problem is really that important. Of course, it can be argued that only the Client can decide if an issue is important or not, but sometimes a second and unbiased opinion can be useful. For example, a survey may be commissioned to delay a decision rather than to actually gather information.

(c) consider whether the Client will make the 'preferred' decision independent of the survey results.

There are many ways of collecting information, and conducting a survey is just one technique amongst many. If the objective is rephrased, a different method of collecting information may prove to be easier and more accurate. *For example, on behalf of a hospital, a Researcher is trying to measure the race and sex of employees to determine if the hospital meets Equal Opportunities legislation. It is possible to send all staff a survey in which they tick the appropriate boxes about their race and sex. Alternatively, it may be possible to examine employment records or for some other hard, objective data to be collected.* This is probably a better way of collecting objective information which avoids the need of conducting a survey.

Now consider the collection of objective information which may be perceived by employees as intrusive and harmful. *A hospital is interested in determining exactly how many hours Researchers spend at work. This is a sensitive issue for staff since the end result could be disciplinary action. It may be possible to record attendance objectively without using a survey, and such methods are more likely to be accurate than a survey.* However, while underhand observation of staff may enable accurate and unbiased assessment, if information is not collected openly and ethically, then the chief result of the exercise will be reduced trust and increased alienation. In this case, it may be that a survey, which contains a consent form and a statement of the objectives of the survey, is in fact a good way to collect the required information.

It is not an overstatement to say that underhand and devious ways of collecting information about employees (even if they are only perceived to be underhand) will always end in disaster. At some point the employees will begin to suspect that they have been deceived and sometimes trust (such as that between management and staff or administrators and practitioners) can be wiped out by a single act. A straightforward and honest approach to information collection is, at the end of the day, the only way of maintaining trust within an organization. A Researcher should therefore understand the strengths and weaknesses of conducting a survey when compared with alternative techniques and the less obvious repercussions of using these methods.

Select, adapt or create?

There are literally thousand of surveys and questionnaires already in existence designed to measure particular beliefs, attitudes and opinions. Once the survey method has been decided upon, it makes sense to spend time determining whether the same issue has been explored in the past by other researchers. It will be far easier to use a questionnaire already in existence, or to adapt a questionnaire, rather than spend time developing one from scratch (see Figure 2, p. 34). It is therefore good practice to create a new survey only as a last resort.

The first place for the Researcher to go to is the library and/or the internet (see Chapter 4 for more information about libraries and the net) to review the literature already in existence.

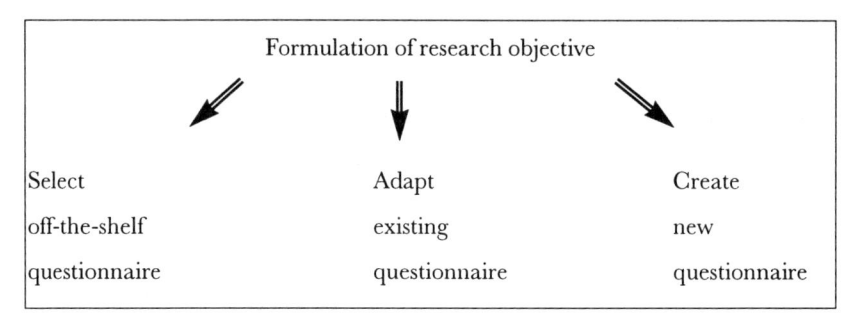

```
                    Formulation of research objective
              ↙                    ↓                    ↘
    Select                      Adapt                      Create
    off-the-shelf               existing                   new
    questionnaire               questionnaire              questionnaire
```

Figure 2. Select, adapt or create

With regard to questionnaires and surveys designed to measure health, the reader is advised to consult the book by McDowell and Newell (1987), which provides a thorough evaluation of current rating scales. Their book describes rating scales already in use in the following areas: (a) functional disability and handicap (b) psychological wellbeing (c) social health (d) quality of life and life satisfaction (e) pain measurement and (f) general health measures. Pearson (1988) provides a good guide to measurement of nurse performance in terms of quality of patient care, the 'nursing audit' and peer review.

Bowling's book *Measuring Disease* (1995) is also an excellent source of questionnaire material associated with the health professions. Her book covers a wide range of health-related questionnaires and provides a lot of background material about their construction, reliability and validity. See Box 2 for a list of the contents of this book.

Box 2

Questionnaires described in *Measuring Disease* (A Bowling, 1995)

This book lists a large number of health-related questionnaires divided up into convenient chapters. It also contains a great deal of useful information about what is known about these questionnaires (reproduced by the kind permission of Open University Press).

1 Health-related quality of life: A discussion of the concept, its use and measurement

Background: The 'quality of life'
What is quality of life and health-related quality of life? A review of the concepts and some attempts at measurement
A concept of health
The public's view of health
Recent interest and developments in measuring health-related quality of life
The need to operationalize health-related quality of life
Quality of life assessment and research on health care outcomes
Utility assessments and quality of life assessments
Generic, domain- and disease-specific measurement scales
Satisfaction with care and outcome
Who should rate quality of life?

2 Cancers

The importance of measuring the quality of life of cancer patients
What has been measured in studies of the quality of life of cancer patients?
What should be measured?
Recommended measurement scales
Review articles on quality of life measurement and cancer
The domain of measurement
The measurement scales
Scales measuring physical functioning, pain and symptoms
Functional status scales used with cancer patients
The Karnofsky Performance Scale
The World Health Organization Functional Scale
The Zubrod Scale (or, the Eastern Cooperative Oncology Group Performance Scale: ECOGP)
Pain scales
The McGill Pain Questionnaire (MPQ)
Other symptom scales
Symptom Distress Scale
Lasry Sexual Functioning Scale for Breast Cancer Patients
Summary of other symptom scales
World Health Organization (WHO) Symptom Checklist
Medical Research Council (MRC) UK Scale
The Qualitator

(contd)

Disease-specific quality of life scales
European Organization for Research on Treatment of Cancer (EORTC) Modular Approach
Rotterdam Symptoms Checklist
Functional Living Index - Cancer (FLIC)
Functional Living Index - Emesis (FLIE)
Cancer Inventory of Problem Situations (CIPS) and the Cancer Rehabilitation Evaluation System (CARES)
Visual Analogue Scales
Spitzer Quality of Life (QL) Index
Linear Analogue Self-Assessment (LASA) Scale
Other visual analogue scales
Ontario Cancer Institute/Royal Marsden Linear Analogue Self-assessment Scale
Padilla Quality of Life (QL) Scale and variants, including the Multi-dimensional Quality of Life Scale - (MQOLS-CA)
Homes and Dickerson
Global Quality of Life Scale (Coates)
Quality of Life Index
Breast Cancer Chemotherapy Questionnaire (BCCQ)
Visual Analogue Scale (VAS) for Bone Marrow Transplant Patients
European Neuroblastoma Study Group Quality of Life Assessment Form - Children (QLAF-C)
Brief Details of Other Scales
Cancer Leukaemia Group B Studies (CALGB)
Ability Index
Burge Quality of Life Severity Scale
Anamnestic Comparative Self-Assessment (ACSA)
World Health Organization Quality of Life Assessment Instrument (WHOQOL)
TWiST
Conclusion

3 Psychiatric conditions and psychological morbidity

Quality of life research and psychiatric and psychological morbidity
Measuring quality of life in institutions
Community indicators of quality of life

Measuring quality of life in individuals: The domain of measurements
Subjective accounts and the value of patient's ratings

The measurement scales

Part I Symptom scales

Background
Symptom questionnaires
Hopkins Symptom Checklist (SCL) and the Symptom Checklist-90
Brief Symptom Inventory (BSI)
Symptom Rating Test (SRT)
Center of Epidemiological Studies of Depression Scale (CES-D)
Rand Depression Screener
Hospital Anxiety and Depression (HAD) Scale
Goldberg's General Health Questionnaire
Beck Depression Inventory
Hamilton Depression Scale
Zung Self-rating Depression Scale
State-Trait Anxiety Inventory (STAI)
Profile of Mood States (POMS)
Scales for children
Conclusion

Part II Quality of life instruments

Condition-specific quality of life scales
Quality of Life Scale (QLS)
Lehman Quality of Life Interview
Lancashire Quality of Life Scale (SBQOL)
Oregon Quality of Life Self-report Questionnaire and Semi-structured
Interview Rating Version
Quality of Life Index for Mental Health (QLI-MH)
Index of Health-related Quality of Life
Piloting of the Health of the Nation Outcome Scales
Team for the Assessment of Psychiatric Services (TAPS) Measures
General Well-being Schedule (GWBS)
Scale for assessing needs
Key Informant Survey Scales
The MRC Needs for Care Assessment

(contd)

Wyke's Assessment of Need Questionnaire
Services Needed, Available, Planned, Offered, Rendered Instrument
Patient Attitude scales
Social Problem Questionnaire
Client Satisfaction Questionnaire (CSQ)
Satisfaction with Life Domain Scale
Conclusion

Part III Role functioning and related instruments

Role functioning, performance and social behaviour scales
Social Functioning Schedule
Social Role Performance Schedule (SRPS)
Social Behaviour Schedule (SBS)
Rehabilitation Evaluation (REHAB)
Social Behaviour Assessment Schedule (SBAS)
WHO Psychiatric Disability Assessment Schedule (WHODAS)
Global Assessment Scale (GAS)
Global Assessment of Functioning Scale (GAFS)
Adjustment and adaptation scales for use with psychiatrically and/or physically ill people
Social Adjustment Scale - II (SAS-II) and Self-report Version
Katz Adjustment Scales
Psychosocial Adjustment to Illness Scale (PAIS)
Global Adjustment to Illness Scale (GAIS)
Acceptance of Illness Scale
Reintegration to Normal Living (RNL) Index
Stress and coping scales for use with psychiatrically and/or physically ill people
Ways of Coping Scale
Health and Daily Living Form
Stress in Life Coping Scale
COPE
Control over Life
Rotter's Internal–External Locus of Control Scale
Multidimensional Health Locus of Control Scales
Conclusion

4 Respiratory conditions

Quality of life in respiratory disease sufferers
The domains of measurement
Measurement scales
Symptom-specific scales: Dyspnoea
The Fletcher Scale and the MRC Dyspnoea Grade and Respiratory Symptoms Questionnaire
Other variations
American Thoracic Society (ATS) Respiratory Questionnaire and Grade of Breathlessness Scale
Horsley Respiratory Symptoms Questionnaire
Summary of other indices of dyspnoea
American Lung Association Severity of Disability (COAD)
Feinstein's Index of Dyspnoea
Severity of Symptoms Visual Analogue Scale (VAS)
Oxygen Cost Diagram
The 6 and 12 Minute Walking Tests and Stair Climbing
Borg Ratio of Perceived Exertion
Mahler Baseline and Transition Dyspnoea Index
Disease-specific quality of life measures
Quality of life assessment in COPD/COAD patients: Disease-specific scales
Guyatt's McMaster Chronic Respiratory Questionnaire (CRQ)
St. George's Respiratory Questionnaire (SGRQ)
Chronic Disease Assessment Tool (CDAT)
Health Outcomes Institute TyPE Scales (HOI-TyPE)-COPD
Quality of life assessment in asthma patients: Disease-specific scales
Asthma Severity Scale
Living with Asthma Questionnaire
Outcome Measures in Ambulatory Care (Asthma and Diabetes) (OMAC)
Health Outcome Institute TyPE Scales (HOL-TyPE) - Asthma Form
Asthma Quality of Life Questionnaire
Asthma Symptom Checklist
Summary of other scales which await full psychometric testing
Asthma Self-efficacy Scale
Attitudes to Asthma Scale
Conclusion

(contd)

5 Neurological conditions

Measuring health-related quality of life in neurology
Cerebrovascular accident (CVA/stroke)
The domains of measurement
Measurement scales
Stroke scales
Rankin Handicap Scale
National Institute of Health Stroke Scale
Canadian Neurological Scale (CNS)
Hemispheric Stroke Scale
Disease-specific measures of quality of life: Functional ability
Barthel Index
Nottingham Extended Activities of Daily Living Questionnaire
Frenchay Activities Index
Rivermead Mobility Index (RMI)
Disease-specific measures of quality of life: Stroke
Health Outcomes Institute TyPE Scales (HOI-TyPE) - Acute Stroke
Kudo Battery for Stroke Patients
Epilepsies
The domains of measurement
What instruments have been used?
Measurement scales
A severity measurement scale
Seizure Severity Scale
Disease-specific quality of life scales: Epilepsy
Washington Psychosocial Inventory
Epilepsy Surgery Inventory
Katz Adjustment Scales (revised for use with epilepsy)
Other
Health-related Quality of Life Model
General test of neurophysiological functioning
Trail-making Test
Wechsler Scales
Wechsler Memory Scale (WMS)
Wechsler Adult Intelligence Scale (WAIS)
Scales for children
Tests for cognitive impairment in elderly people
Abbreviated Mental Test Score (AMTS)

Mini-Mental State Examination (MMSE)
Mental Status Questionnaire (MSQ)
Older Americans' Resources and Services Schedule (OARS) mental health measures
Brief Cognitive Functioning Scale (SIP sub-scale)
Geriatric Mental State (GMS) and Comprehensive Assessment and Referral Evaluation (CARE)
Conclusion

6 Rheumatological conditions

Quality of life in people with joint disorders
The domains of measurement
The measurement scales
Disease severity and functional classifications
Disease-specific scales: Physical functioning
Stanford Arthritis Center Health Assessment Questionnaire (HAQ)
Arthritis Impact Measurement Scales (AIMS)
Functional Status Index (FSI)
Western Ontario and McMaster Universities Arthritis Index (WOMAC)
Office of Population Censuses and Surveys (OPCS) Disability Scale
Rheumatoid Arthritis (RA) Impact on the Homemaker Questionnaire
Broader disease-specific quality of life scales
MACTAR (McMaster-Toronto Arthritis) Patient Function Preference Questionnaire
Hornquist's Quality of Life Status and Change Scale
Schedule for the Evaluation of Individual Quality of Life (SEIQoL)
Health Outcomes Institute TyPE (HOI-TyPE) - Joint Conditions
Rand Joint Problems Battery
Summaries of the scales
Arthritis Helplessness Index (AHI)
EURIDISS (European Research on Incapacitating Diseases and Social Support)
Conclusion

7 Cardiovascular diseases

Heart Disease
Trends in measuring quality of life in people with heart disease

(contd)

Most and least frequently used indicators
What should be measured?
The domains of measurement
The measurement scales
Categorizations and measures of physical activity
New York Heart Association Functional Classification Scale
Olsson Ranking Scale
Canadian Cardiovascular Society Functional Classification for Angina Pectoris
Specific Activity Scale (SAS)
Rankin Handicap Scale
Symptom questionnaires
Dyspnoea scales
Fletcher Questionnaire and the Rose (WHO) Questionnaires: The London School of Hygiene Dyspnoea Questionnaire and Cardiovascular Questionnaire (Angina of Effort)
Other Scales
Feinstein's Index of Dyspnoea
Ratio Property Scale
Disease-specific quality of life scales: Heart disease
Health Outcomes Institute TyPE Scales (HOI-TyPE) - Angina
Rand Congestive Heart Failure (Shortness of breath/Enlarged heart/heart failure) Battery and Rand Chest Pain (Angina) Battery
Guyatt's Chronic Heart Failure Questionnaire (CHQ)
Ferrans and Powers' Quality of Life Index (CARDIAC)
Rehabilitation Questionnaire
Circulatory disease
Trends in measuring quality of life in people with circulatory disease - Hypertension
What should be measured?
Disease-specific quality of life scales: Hypertension
Palmer's Symptom Checklist and Battery
Health Outcomes Institute TyPE Scales (HOI-TyPE) - Hypertension
Bulpitt's Hypertension Questionnaire and Batteries
Quality of Life Impairment Scale - Hypertension
Rand Health Insurance Study Blood Pressure Battery
Conclusion

8 Other disease- and condition-specific scales

Other developments in the measurement of disease-specific quality of life
Health Outcomes Institute TyPE Scales (HOI-TyPE)
Popular generic measures used to supplement disease-specific scales
Disease-specific measures of quality of life
Diabetes
Outcome Measures in Ambulatory Care (Asthma and Diabetes) (OMAC)
Diabetes Impact Measurement Scales (DIMS)
Quality of Life Status and Change (QLSC)
Health Outcomes Institute TyPE Scales (HOI-TyPE) - Diabetes
Rand Diabetes Mellitus Battery
Diabetes Quality of Life Measure (DQOL)
Renal disease
Functional classification
The use of generic scales and domain-specific batteries
Haemodialysis Quality of Life Questionnaire (HQLQ)
Leicester Uraemic Symptom Scale (LUSS)
Quality of Life Assessment
Bowel diseases
Inflammatory Bowel Disease Questionnaire (IBIQ)
Rand Surgical Condition Battery: Haemorrhoids
Human Immunodeficiency Virus (HIV) and Acquired Immune Deficiency Syndrome (AIDS)
HIV Overview of Problems-Evaluation System (HOPES)
AIDS Health Assessment Questionnaire
Varicose veins
Varicose Veins Questionnaire
Rand Surgical Conditions Battery: Varicose Veins
Back pain
Clinical Back Pain Questionnaire
Children
Elderly people
A popular core (generic) measure for use in disease-specific studies in adults: The short Form-36 (SF-36)

Those Researchers who wish to design measures of work experience would do well to consult the excellent compendium and review of nearly 250 measures by Cook, Hepworth, Wall and Warr (1981).

The advantages of using off-the-shelf questionnaires may include:

- published and good psychometric properties
- reliance on work conducted by previous Researchers
- possible availability of a manual
- addition to the body of research knowledge in a direct way
- comparison to norms already established
- easy to use once selected.

and the disadvantages may include that it is:

- expensive to buy
- should not be copied without permission of the copyright holder
- too general for use in the way that the Researcher wants to use it
- not appropriate for use in this new situation.

However the advantages of creating a new questionnaire include:

- specificity in the sense that the questionnaire was designed directly for the use that it is being put to

and the disadvantages include:

- possible waste of resources, time and effort
- need to conduct a pilot study
- need to develop knowledge of the psychometric properties.

Can the survey be completed within the time frame?

The Client is unlikely to be fully aware that surveys take a long time to complete, so the Researcher must make it clear that meaningful conclusions cannot be drawn within short time frames and that cutting too many corners to achieve results quickly is likely to produce invalid conclusions.

Example: A Client needs to determine attitudes to euthanasia within the health professions to answer a ministerial enquiry. The Client asks the Researcher to conduct a survey and report back within two months. Two months may seem a long time but the nature of the subject suggests the need for sensitivity and research by experts to determine the right kind of survey questions for such a large and complex subject. This kind of survey would require large amounts of time and resources to conduct and so, under normal conditions, valid conclusions concerning a project such as this could not be drawn within two months. In fact a project of this type may well take six months or even longer.

Consider the risks of postponing the survey

This is a question that too few ask, but which all should consider. It is unwise to postpone a survey continually until there is no time left in which to perform it, or major problems cannot be corrected in time. With the benefit of hindsight, it is quite often the case that Researchers and Clients have a good perception of the risks that were attached to a project once it has been completed. At the time, however, it is much more likely resources will be under-allocated and insufficient time will have been spent in the planning stages of the project. It is important for the Researcher to have adequate time to undertake the project. Postponing the start of a survey until the last moment is usually a recipe for disaster.

Get a written contract

Most of the time Researchers will find that they are working with colleagues who are reasonably honest in their approach to work. They mean what they say, and their word is their bond. However a Researcher does not have to be in the business of writing and administering surveys and questionnaires for long to come across colleagues who have somewhat lower standards of behaviour. Unfortunately it is not always possible to identify these people before beginning the work. Therefore it is crucial to have a written contract concerning the work that will be done. Clearly the type of contract depends upon whether the Researcher is external or internal to the organization, the nature of the work being undertaken and the relationship between Researcher and the Client. In Box 3 we present an example of a general contract between a Client and an external consultancy.

Box 3

Example terms of business

All Researchers in the business of conducting surveys for Clients should get a contract as this is useful in describing the business relationship between the parties. Hopefully such contracts will be put in the drawer and never read again after they have been signed. However, very rarely, a contract may need to be referred to in the case of serious misunderstandings between the Client and the Researcher.

There are many types of contracts and we provide an example of a very general one that sets out the relationship between a client and a consultancy. There would normally be a specific proposal to undertake the work as well as this document. Thanks to Mike Wellin of Behaviour Transformation Ltd. for supplying the contract.

1. Delivering client results

All consultancy assignments undertaken by Behaviour Transformation Ltd focus on the achievement of specific objectives and results which have been agreed beforehand with the client. These objectives and targeted results are stated in a formal proposal document or letter. The proposal document or letter and these terms of business constitute an offer to perform the assignment which has as its purpose the achievement of stated objectives and results.

If the client desires to change the stated objectives and targeted results once an assignment has commenced these must be advised in writing. Behaviour Transformation Ltd will do its best to achieve any proposed revised objectives within the assignment terms, but reserves the right to alter either the price or delivery terms for the assignment if it deems this necessary.

All completion time estimates for proposals are based on best estimates. These are dependent on Behaviour Transformation resources, and client cooperation, and both of these may be subject to factors not in our control. Behaviour Transformation will, however, take all reasonable steps to ensure that completion dates where given are achieved.

Behaviour Transformation operate a client and project management system. This involves the planning and regular monitoring of consultant and client activities involved in delivering an assignment, so that these have the best possible impact on the achievement of client results. All assignments are supervised, and it is a condition of our engagement that the client permit supervision and quality reviews whether explicitly stated in the proposal or not. We cannot accept liability for any losses that are not reasonably foreseeable on acceptance of the proposal, or for any indirect or consequential losses, including loss of revenue, anticipated profits and claims by third parties.

In the event of client concerns about a project, these should be raised directly with the project manager. The project manager is: _____.

Behaviour Transformation reserve the right to use suitably qualified associates or sub-contracted personnel. In all such cases, however, such personnel are under the direct control of a Behaviour Transformation project manager.

If during the course of an assignment a need is identified for additional or ancillary activities or services not specified in the original proposal, their use will be subject to agreement with the client before any additional expenditure is incurred.

2. Client collaboration

All investigations, assessments and recommendations in any proposal, report or letter are made in good faith, and on the basis of the information made available by the client. Their achievement depends on the full cooperation of the client and the client's staff. In consequence, no statement in any proposal, presentation, report or letter is deemed to be a warranty of achievable results.

The client will be responsible for the provision of suitable office premises and services, together with such information, management and employee time and specific facilities as may be reasonably required to fulfil our obligations, whether defined or not in the proposal. The client will use all reasonable endeavours to respond quickly and positively to requests for information, consultation, decisions, and approvals.

3. Charges and costs
An estimate of our consultancy charges for this assignment are

(contd)

provided in the proposal document/letter attached. These costs are for all consultant time spent on the assignment, whether at the client's premises or not, as well as any direct administrative costs. Travelling and subsistence expenses for our staff, and other incidental expenses including venue costs for running events connected with the assignment will be recharged at cost. VAT will also be added to the cost of consultant time, travelling and other expenses.

The proposal together with these terms of business constitute an offer to perform the consultancy assignment at a particular price. The estimated charges will not be exceeded without the client's prior agreement.

4. Confidentiality

It is normal for our work to involve access to client confidential information. Except for the purposes of this assignment, neither party shall without the prior written consent of the other use, exploit, divulge or disclose to third parties any commercial or confidential information, business systems or methodologies, proprietary systems or application programs of the other, which may be communicated or gained in connection with this assignment. This restriction shall cease to apply to the divulging of information which:

1) Is in or later comes into the public domain, other than by breach of the foregoing paragraph
2) Is in the possession of the recipient, with the full right to disclose it, prior to receiving it from the other party
3) Is independently received by the recipient from a third party with the full right to disclose it
4) Either party is obliged by law to disclose

We shall not announce publicly that we are providing services to the client unless the client consents in advance to such disclosure. No press releases concerning the assignment will be made without both parties' consent.

The copyright of all reports, and data submitted to clients will remain the property of Behaviour Transformation until payment of the final invoice, when copyright will transfer to the client.

(Reproduced by kind permission of Mike Wellin of Behaviour Transformation Ltd)

Funding for the project

The final stage of planning the survey is to assess cost and funding implications. Assessing cost is a difficult component of best practice in survey design. The best advice is to look at the cost of previous surveys of a similar nature. In assessing the cost, the Researcher should not forget all the specific stages that are needed to undertake a survey. For example, data entry into the computer can be time-consuming and easily overlooked. Another component of data entry is labelling of all the columns in the software spreadsheet. If it is done properly, as it should be so that adequate records are kept, it can take several hours to do. The Researcher should also make sure that appropriate funding is available from the Client and that external contractors (for example, professional Interviewers) understand the nature of their responsibilities and relationships with the research team and the Client. It is important that these ancillary people know how and when they will be paid.

The Researcher will need to assess the cost of the following aspects of a project, among others:

(a) Development of the survey design
 – Defining the objective
 – Developing the theory/model to be tested
 – Obtaining practical information about what the Client requires
 – Writing the items
 – Designing the assessment method
 – Trial of the survey
(b) Administration of the survey
 – Printing of survey
 – Delivery of survey
 – Collection of completed survey
(c) Data entry of results into computer
(d) Data analysis
(e) Writing of report
(f) Presenting results
(g) Other costly components such as liaising with staff, travel, meetings to agree items, etc.

Do not underestimate the political dimension

The best way for a Researcher to avoid having a project scuppered by red tape and political infighting is to remember the politics of large organizations. As various people examine the project proposal, the Researcher may find that attempts are made to block its progress. Although the Researcher must never forget the ethics, it is important to market the project in the right way to the right people, and to persevere so that these problems are overcome. Only then will the project progress.

For example, a Researcher finds that the cooperation of senior managers is required so that a survey can be administered to their staff. One of them refuses to cooperate, saying that 'surveys are a waste of time' and that the staff are too busy. How can a point-blank refusal by a key person to cooperate be overcome? There are several ways to do this:

(a) Effective marketing. Sell the project (ethically and honestly) so that the manager sees the reasons why the survey is important (which presumably it is or the research would not have been commissioned).

(b) Often these blanket refusals are used because the person concerned has a hidden agenda. The Researcher should organize a meeting and attempt to identify the problems. By dealing directly with these issues, it may be much easier to get the cooperation of key staff.

However, it is important not to cut corners in order to achieve the project aims. When barriers are placed in the way of the project's success, best practice demands that official procedures are followed and not ignored. The costs of ignoring the rules of how a project should be conducted can easily outweigh the benefits. Once the objective is clearly defined the Researcher should make sure that it receives the necessary authorization, and quite often this stage is lengthy and frustrating. Best practice is to persevere and obtain authorization rather than deliberately avoid authorization (for example, by performing the survey unofficially). Ultimately the over-enthusiastic Researcher will be very badly exposed if the results of an unauthorized survey are poorly received.

For example, an administrative officer wishes to send out a survey to all the radiographers in the hospital. The administrative officer could get official authorization and contact the radiographers through official channels. On the other hand, the administrative officer may know someone in personnel who will hand over the personal details of the radiographers so that they can be contacted directly. Such a plan may be easier, but it is not best practice. Best practice dictates that the Researcher go through official channels.

Summary

The Researcher should:

(a) understand the appropriateness and ethics of the Client's survey. The Researcher should be prepared to return to the Client when unhappy about the objectives, and may need to refer problems to an ethics committee.
(b) understand what the conclusions of the survey may be, what its uses will be, and who will be in charge of summarizing and disseminating the results.
(c) establish that there is a genuine reason for undertaking the survey work and that the survey can be finished within the agreed amount of time.
(d) obtain necessary authorization and follow official channels.
(e) get a written contract.
(f) properly cost the project.
(g) be prepared for the almost inevitable political dimension to the project.

Chapter 4
Researching the problem

Introduction

Once the Researcher has decided to undertake the survey work, the next step is to gain an overview of how the problem is to be tackled. Survey design is almost always more complex than originally envisaged, and so the competence of the Researcher to undertake a difficult project needs to be considered by both the Client and the Researcher. The Client has a clear interest in making sure that the Researcher is competent enough to do the job. However, this is also true of the Researcher. Having said that, some Researchers may well need to overcome initial nervousness about their competence even though they are extremely able.

Even for surveys of small scope, the Researcher may still need to turn to experts and books to understand the area of the survey, and to ensure it conforms with current theory (see Box 4). With a survey of broader scope (e.g. to measure the culture of a health profession), the Researcher is likely to need to turn to an expert for advice.

For example, on the face of it a survey to identify whether patients are satisfied with the comfort of their beds appears to be well within the competence of anyone. The simple question: 'How comfortable is your bed?' seems obvious. Or is it? This question establishes the level of satisfaction with the bed that is currently being used by the patient. However, a better objective of the survey would be to identify the aspects of a bed that are most important in determining patient satisfaction. Questions need therefore to be asked about what it is that makes a bed comfortable. An apparently simple survey has suddenly become more complex.

It is also possible that patients with different ailments and patients who are in hospital for different lengths of time will have preferences for different types of bed.

It would then be necessary to collect sufficiently large samples of patients in these categories to determine whether this is the case. It becomes clear that what at first seems an easy project is becoming much more complex by the minute. Does the Researcher have the competence to conduct this survey? (Equally, as discussed in the first section, does the Client really have the will to do anything about such a survey anyway? Perhaps as these issues are explored, it becomes clear that the Client does not believe in patient comfort to the extent of having different beds for different patients!)

Box 4

Why thorough research is necessary

Try this interesting exercise. List all the types of alternative medicine that you can before looking at the table below, where you will find an example questionnaire about alternative medicine that has been used by Professor Adrian Furnham after an extensive amount of research. Compare your list with this list and you may well be surprised at what you have left out. What about the therapies that you have listed and that Furnham has left out? Is the list below adequate and are the therapies correctly labelled? Or is it inadequate? Without research it is unlikely that the whole domain of possible items would be included in the questionnaire. Furnham's questionnaire asks Respondents to tick appropriate boxes for alternative medicine practices that they have heard about, have tried, or would try.

	Heard about	Have tried	Would try
Acupuncture	[ ]	[ ]	[ ]
Alexander technique	[ ]	[ ]	[ ]
Anthroposophical medicine	[ ]	[ ]	[ ]
Applied kinesiology	[ ]	[ ]	[ ]
Aromatherapy	[ ]	[ ]	[ ]
Art therapy	[ ]	[ ]	[ ]
Auricular therapy	[ ]	[ ]	[ ]
Chiropody	[ ]	[ ]	[ ]
Chiropractic	[ ]	[ ]	[ ]
Clinical ecology and allergy	[ ]	[ ]	[ ]

(contd)

Colonic hydrotherapy	[ ]	[ ]	[ ]
Colour therapy	[ ]	[ ]	[ ]
Crystal/gem therapy	[ ]	[ ]	[ ]
Dowsing	[ ]	[ ]	[ ]
Eye therapy	[ ]	[ ]	[ ]
Hair therapy	[ ]	[ ]	[ ]
Healing	[ ]	[ ]	[ ]
Herbalism	[ ]	[ ]	[ ]
Homeopathy	[ ]	[ ]	[ ]
Horticultural therapy	[ ]	[ ]	[ ]
Hypnosis/hypnotherapy	[ ]	[ ]	[ ]
Iridology	[ ]	[ ]	[ ]
Magnet therapy	[ ]	[ ]	[ ]
Massage	[ ]	[ ]	[ ]
Music therapy	[ ]	[ ]	[ ]
Naturopathy	[ ]	[ ]	[ ]
Osteopathy	[ ]	[ ]	[ ]
Polarity therapy	[ ]	[ ]	[ ]
Radionics	[ ]	[ ]	[ ]
Structural integration therapy	[ ]	[ ]	[ ]
Yoga therapy	[ ]	[ ]	[ ]

Let us take another example. *A survey has been commissioned to investigate how staff at a big city hospital come to work. The client is interested in knowing the means of transport, the cost and the time taken. Initially a simple problem, the scale of the project becomes very complex as the Researcher investigates. Some staff will use multiple means on the same trip (e.g. car to railway station, train, then the underground and then walk); some staff will use obscure means of transport (e.g. roller skates, river boat and perhaps even aircraft or international train). Moreover, the means of transport may well vary depending on the weather (e.g. in summer, people may walk across a river bridge whereas in winter they might take a bus). Designing a survey that fully describes how staff get to hospital is clearly not as simple as it seems.*

Researchers should be prepared to rely on the assistance of experts (for instance, and most commonly, in the data analysis), but they should not become overly reliant on the experts. Experts should never be used to correct sloppy or shoddy work. For example, poor use of English when constructing questionnaire items or poorly designed rating scales reflect lack of effort and commitment on the part of the Researcher. Moreover, work needs to be a learning experience and Researchers who always ask for assistance will also be reducing their chances for self-development.

It is also useful to have other books on survey material as further reference. We have tried to make this book a relatively fresh and interesting approach to the use of surveys and questionnaires within the health professions. More general survey books that we recommend and have not directly referenced elsewhere include Babbie, 1973; Fink and Cosec, 1985; Foddy, 1995; Moser and Kalton, 1971; Oppenheim, 1992; Rosenberg, 1968 and Schuman and Presser, 1981. It is likely that your library will have at least one of these texts and we are sure that they will provide a useful supplement to our book. Oppenheim (1992) is widely considered to be an excellent source.

Developing knowledge about the research question

The Researcher can develop knowledge of the research question by:

(a) Becoming familiar with the subject and being forced to 'go public' in some way with this information. The Researcher could try writing a review of the subject areas, doing a seminar or other presentation with colleagues whose viewpoint is respected. If a Researcher is able to tell others about the project, the chances are that he or she understands the subject area.
(b) Widening the field of experience. The Researcher should read broadly from different subject areas. There may be many other Researchers who are facing similar research problems, or who have already solved them. Contact and discussion provides an alternative and better perspective of the research question.
(c) Avoiding being trapped in a line of thought by assuming that the answer to the research question is obvious. Very little in survey design is obvious when the subject is thought through quite deeply. The Researcher needs to keep an open mind when investigating the problem and needs to be prepared to change direction when necessary.
(d) Avoiding trying to answer questions that cannot be answered. The nature of the research question may mean that there is no clear answer, or that answer is too difficult for the Researcher to

obtain using a survey or questionnaire. *For example, a Researcher is asked to conduct a survey on the causes of cot death within the local population. In general, a survey will not establish a direct causal relationship between two or more variables (unless external measures are used within an experimental study) so hypotheses along these lines should be avoided. However, a survey might reveal interesting trends and possibilities for further research.*

The literature review

Possibly the most influential factor (apart from the Client) that will decide the way the research is conducted is the literature review itself. In general, the major part of any serious piece of work is the literature review. This is central to the whole research process and is a critical and comprehensive review of what has been written on the topic. It is therefore an attempt to collect, read, summarize and learn from all the salient research that has been previously undertaken in the subject area. It ensures that you do not 'reinvent the wheel' or fall into traps that others have already come across.

The literature review is definitely not something that is done early and then forgotten. Instead it is a continuous process that carries on throughout the research programme. It is likely to change the direction and usefulness of the research according to the particular stage that has been reached. Of course the main literature review will take place at the start of the project, but expect about 30 or 40% of the total time available for a serious research project to be taken up in reviewing the literature. As the research proceeds, the Researcher should expect to re-examine the literature to answer specific questions about methodology, or perhaps to determine whether the results that have been obtained were satisfactorily explained by others at an earlier time. By doing this, the Researcher should establish that the present study is not just a repeat of past work (which may therefore make this investigation redundant), and should learn how to avoid pitfalls that previous Researchers have encountered. A good literature review tells the Researcher how people have thought about and dealt with the problem in the past.

The preliminary search of the Researcher will be centred on the following questions:

(a) Obtaining a general understanding of the relevant literature concerning the survey topic.
(b) Precise definition of the research objectives.
(c) How to test the hypotheses that may be developed from the research objective.
(d) The advantages and disadvantages of the research method that has been chosen.
(e) Understanding how to measure the variables that the Client is interested in.
(f) Developing a clear theoretical rationale for the research.

Box 5

Using libraries to review the literature

Most reports containing a survey begin with a literature review which explains why the present research is interesting and important in the context of research that has previously been conducted on this topic. This means that the reader of the report does not have to take for granted the authority of the author to conduct the research; qualified readers can determine for themselves whether the Researcher has made a strong case in the report for the conclusions that are drawn. To be able to write a literature review, a Researcher must make use of a library, the internet or some other database. In fact, however, the Researcher needs to make good use of a library right from the start of the project so that the research problem can be properly understood and refined.

For this type of research libraries come in four types - academic, public, hospital based and professional society based. Academic libraries are usually well stocked with highly informative and authoritative texts. This type of library also contains scientific journals featuring the latest research within a particular area. There can, however, be two problems with academic libraries. First, they are daunting. The sheer amount of research material is often overwhelming and the texts are often written in the particular jargon of the discipline with which the book or journal is concerned. As a result a simple survey can become far too complex. The second problem with academic libraries is one of access. Unless the Researcher is a student or a member of staff, it is not very easy to gain admission. At

(contd)

the very least, there will be a charge. Public libraries are more accessible and usually carry a broader range of titles, although the number of titles in one particular area will tend to be limited. Some hospitals or similar institutions may have their own libraries for use by health professionals. This can be a useful and convenient first start for health-related surveys, especially as these libraries may be able to obtain books and other material by borrowing them from other libraries. The fourth possibility is to gain access to a library controlled by a professional society. For example, the Royal College of Nursing in London has a very wide collection of books relevant to that particular discipline. These professional libraries tend to be very specialized to a particular profession but also very complete. If the Researcher is a member of that society then these libraries can also be very accessible, providing that the library is within a reasonable distance. The Researcher should decide, according to the level of complexity of the research project, which type of library is best.

In most libraries the Researcher will find:

(a) Books, generally arranged according to a subject-based cataloguing method.
(b) Journals, newspapers and professional magazines.
(c) A catalogue which lists the material that the library stocks by author, title and by subject area. Many libraries have computerized catalogues which make the search very easy after just a short amount of practice.

In academic libraries, the Researcher will also find:

(d) Abstracts containing a brief summary of recent research work, under various classifications. Many abstracts are now computerized, making the search for material very straightforward. 'Nursing Abstracts', for example, lists and describes a wide range of research on nursing.
(e) Annual review journals.
(f) The opportunity to get access to books held by other libraries by means of an Inter-library loan.

Tricks for quickly identifying the best books or articles for the research include:

Researching the problem

> (a) Using computerized databases of abstracts. This is the best technique for obtaining a full list of relevant literature but is not the best technique for the Researcher who wants a less in-depth knowledge of the literature.
> (b) Browsing the bookshelf that is most closely associated with a particular subject area.
> (c) Browsing relevant journals (certainly good for obtaining a feel for a particular area).
> (d) Searching key words.
> (e) Getting the latest relevant publications and working backwards through all the salient literature.

To summarize this important section, the Researcher should always perform a thorough review of the literature; expect the review to be time-consuming but genuinely interesting (for the novice also relatively daunting); expect to review the literature over the span of the whole research project as it is essential to be up-to-date; and use the literature review as something that is central to the whole research project and can be used to answer fundamental questions about the objectives, the 'how', 'what', 'when' and where'.

Advances on the literature review

Meta-analysis has become a popular (but advanced) research method for summarizing the results of past research. The advantage of the method is that it provides a succinct summary of vast amounts of conflicting results. This is particularly useful if there are dozens of separate studies that seem to provide no clear picture about a given area of research.

Meta-analysis is conceptually a simple process that involves collecting the desired descriptive statistics (e.g. correlations, means and other values) from all the available studies. The first thing to do with these data is to present them in the form of a table. This is a valuable addition to a literature review but it can be taken several steps further.

The average of these descriptive statistics and a measure of their variability is taken, due consideration being given to sampling error and other artefacts that may be found in the data. If the mean is more than about two standard deviations from zero, then it is reasonable to conclude that there is a positive relationship. *For example, in a large review of the way assessment centres work Gaugler, Rosenthal, Thornton and Bentson (1987) noted that the range of validities of assessment centres in the literature varied from −0.25 to +0.78. Gaugler* et al. *used meta-analysis to determine both average predictive validity and the causes of the variation that have been reported. The results obtained by Gaugler* et al. *showed that assessment centres had reasonable predictive validity (mean = 0.37). Examination of possible moderating variables indicated that higher validities were found when:*

(a) The criterion was a measure of potential rather than actual performance
(b) Percentage of female assessors was high
(c) Several evaluation methods were used
(d) Assessors were psychologists rather than managers
(e) Peer evaluation was used
(f) Sound methodology was used.

Validity was unaffected by:

(a) Age of assessees
(b) Amount of feedback
(c) Amount of assessor training
(d) Amount of observation
(e) Percentage of minority assessees
(f) Amount of criterion contamination.

You can see that the results of hundreds of studies involving assessment centres, which would have been very difficult to summarize by means of a literature review, have been succinctly listed in just a few lines. Meta-analysis is not without faults as a methodology, but it does offer the advanced Researcher a powerful method for summarizing a complex subject area.

Box 6

Using the internet to research a topic

The internet, or world wide web, offers an interesting alternative to the library as a method of research. There are various search engines (software that searches the web for key words) to make

Researching the problem

> browsing easy, or the Researcher may already know of websites specializing in the area of interest. It is also possible to join forums and interest groups that enable communication between interested parties. All this provides a rich seam of material for the Researcher to exploit.
>
> Two words of warning are required with regard to the web. First, it is very easy to be misled by a professional-looking website into thinking that your contacts are more knowledgeable than they actually are. Do not accept incorrect and erroneous information from biased individuals. If everything on the web were true, the world we live in would be far more interesting than it actually is! Second, do not be swamped by too much information. It is not uncommon to be provided with thousands of interesting possibilities to look at when entering common search items. The Researcher needs to be very specific and expert at searching the web to extract relevant information.
>
> Access to the web is through an internet service provider and you will need a computer and a modem. Your local newsagent will probably stock an internet magazine listing local internet service providers.

Understanding the practice

It is not enough to have an understanding of the theory when designing a survey. Chances are that the Researcher will be a relative outsider to the ways things are done, i.e. the 'culture' of the particular occupational group of interest. The Researcher needs to determine what is current practice both within and outside the group of interest. By talking to subject experts, he or she will be able to develop a feel for the correct expressions and phrases that are important to those knowledgeable about the subject. At this stage it is the general advice that is important, so the Researcher should not get too involved with details.

For example, a senior executive at a large hospital is interested in determining how to get local people involved in fundraising. The Researcher needs to know in general terms what the hospital already does to promote itself to the public (e.g. getting involved with the local community, charity events, open days), and what other organizations do. From this practical perspective, the Researcher will be able to develop some ideas of how the hospital could sell itself better.

Summary

To gain a good understanding of the issues involved in the design of the survey or questionnaire, the Researcher should:

(a) Obtain relevant background information on the subject.
(b) Read professional publications and research the area by using the world wide web, for example.
(c) Contact the appropriate professional body for advice.
(d) Be prepared to make the project simpler in its objectives, or pass the work on to an expert in the field.
(e) Avoid using experts as shortcuts or as excuses for doing poor or shoddy work.
(f) Talk to the practitioners in external or similar organizations.
(g) Be open and able to learn from experiences about the correct way of expressing information.

Part 2
The general survey design

Chapter 5
An overview of the design

Introduction

By now the Researcher will have realized that there are many issues to be considered when planning a survey. However this is not the end of it by any means. Before deciding on the type of survey (postal, interview, telephone, etc.) it is necessary to give some thought to the survey or questionnaire design. This refers to the way in which the general design of the survey is controlled, or organized, by the Researcher. There are two main types of simple design to consider:

1. Non-experimental descriptive approach
(a) cross-sectional (e.g. surveys of several subsets of the population at particular points in time)
(b) longitudinal (e.g. annually for 5 years).

2. Experimental and quasi-experimental approach (e.g. a sample split into an experimental and a control group)

The main difference between the experimental and non-experimental approach is in the type of conclusion that can be drawn once the survey has been completed. Many types of survey set out to describe how things are at a certain period of time or how things change over time. This is all well and good until Researchers want to draw causal inferences from their research. *For example, descriptive research may set out to measure patient morale over a period of time within a hospital. This provides useful management information but does not tell the Researcher why morale increases or decreases. Only by careful design of a study involving known differences between groups (for example, experimental versus control groups) can causal inferences be determined.*

Often survey and questionnaire studies will fall somewhere in between these two extreme forms of design, since experimental research is impractical for many problems. Quasi-experimental designs are pragmatic and are usually the ethical alternatives that can make a good compromise when seeking to discover causal explanations.

Non-experimental descriptive approach

Cross-sectional designs

The cross-sectional approach is the most common type of design used in survey and questionnaire research. With this design, data are collected at a single point in time, usually across representative groups of the population. The groups may consist of sub-sets of a single population (e.g. different departments, different types of patients, etc.) and is a useful type of design when the survey has the objective of measuring opinion or attitudes at some predetermined time. Good examples of this kind of survey are those conducted before or directly after a major change, or when a specific answer is required at some specific time. Cross-sectional surveys are easy to perform, and since they relate to an immediate situation, they provide an opportunity for people to react (i.e. take positive action or have a change of mind). However, if the situation is changing rapidly, the data may soon become outdated.

For example, prior to making changes in the structure of allowances paid to health workers, it was first decided to use a survey to determine levels of satisfaction with the present allowances. A representative cross-section of each major group of health workers was therefore chosen to take part in the survey.

In a second example, before investing a large sum of money in parental suites for the baby care unit, the Client decided to conduct a survey to see how many parents would stay overnight if they had the chance.

The most simple cross-sectional design is when data are collected from just one sample, or from several samples that differ in many ways. Such designs are useful for descriptive purposes only, and it is difficult to infer causality without making major assumptions. When making such assumptions it is all too easy to draw conclusions about causality that reflect one's own biases.

Since cross-sectional designs also do not measure events over two or more periods of time, differences over time cannot be used to determine possible causality. The only way causality may be inferred from a cross-sectional design is by comparing responses from two or more groups of individuals who differ in just one major way (for example, patients undergoing behaviour therapy versus patients undergoing psychoanalysis). The assumption is that if all the other differences between the groups are minimal then this major difference must account for differences in survey or questionnaire responses between the groups. Just how big this assumption is depends on how easy it is to obtain representative groups that differ in just the way defined by the Researcher. In reality there may be gender, age and many other variations between the groups as well as in the differences defined by the Researcher. *For example, to examine the relationship between hypertension and lifestyle of two types of patient, two groups might be chosen, as alike as possible, except that the individuals in one of the groups have high blood pressure. The survey would then aim to discover whether there were any significant differences in lifestyle that could lead to the identification of the factors causing hypertension.*

Sometimes it is possible to compare results from an experimental group with already established norms that are known (such as previously collected average scores). It may be necessary to survey only the experimental group when comparative data are already in existence. For example, an established survey is chosen and given to the group of interest. The results are compared with those previously designated as the 'norm' for this survey, and differences are noted. These differences are then considered to be the result of whatever makes the experimental group 'special'. Normative designs are relatively cheap and easy to run. However, if there are numerous differences between the experimental and the comparison groups, accuracy and validity of conclusions may be severely reduced. *For example, the health professions are worried about poor recruitment to one area of nursing. The objective of the survey is therefore to obtain information about why people do not want to join that particular area. This may be achieved by conducting a survey on existing members of the profession and comparing their results with known norms of nurses who have similar but different jobs. The survey may reveal that working hours and job satisfaction are far higher in the area of nursing of interest compared with the norm number of hours worked by nurses in other areas. Readers may then conclude that the long working day is an important reason for* the poor recruitment of nurses into this particular specialization, on the assumption that increased job satisfaction cannot be related to low recruitment.

It is important that the norms are sufficiently large, not dated and are relevant for the comparison to be useful. If there are uncertainties about the norm group, then it is difficult to make firm conclusions about the group in which you are interested. For example, mothers are especially proud to compare their babies against norm tables and state that their little bundle of joy is in the 90th percentile. This is fine if the norm tables were compiled recently, but if they are quite old most babies born today would probably be in the high percentile range simply because babies are much heavier now than in the past. Moreover the norms must generally have been collected across the same items and in the same manner, and sometimes this kind of information is not available.

Another problem with norms is that they are not always readily transferable across nationalities. Many questionnaires originate in the United States, for example. In itself this is not a bad thing, but the norms reported in the test manuals may not be appropriate for other nationalities. If stereotypes are to be believed, the dangers of using the wrong norms are clear. For example, it seems distinctly likely that the Americans and the British do not share the same personalities. Perhaps Americans are more enthusiastic and naive but less sceptical and cynical than the British.

Longitudinal designs

In contrast to cross-sectional designs, longitudinal designs have the objective of measuring changes of opinion, so that data are collected over a period of time rather than at one specific point in time. There are three variations of longitudinal designs:

Trend designs

A group is selected from a population that has undergone a shared experience for a limited time. This involvement is subsequently repeated by fresh populations at regular intervals as new groups undergo that shared experience. *For example, consider a class of candidates entering physiotherapy school. A survey of race and sex composition might be taken of a sample from the class in the first year. A similar survey could then be conducted on the new classes in the same year over succeeding years as new groups enter the physiotherapy school. Thus, a trend in the ability of the health professions to work towards equal opportunities could be established.*

Cohort designs

A group, selected from people who have undergone a shared experience as described above, is surveyed at selected intervals after the experience. With a cohort design, the composition of the group is not constant, e.g. the group might be selected randomly for each survey. In other words, whilst the trend design examines effects on new groups of people that undergo the same experience, the cohort design looks at effects on the same group of people as they progress from that shared experience. However, it may not be exactly the same people who are surveyed as time progresses; instead it will be a selection of people that varies for each survey. *For example, after a new method had been introduced for training nurses, the nurses' developing skills were monitored by examining randomly chosen groups of that first cohort over the next few years. These skills were then compared against nurses who had been trained using the more traditional method.*

Panel designs

This is similar to the cohort design except that the group composition remains constant every time the survey is administered, i.e. the individuals initially selected are re-surveyed at particular intervals. This design has the advantage that elements of random error are reduced. However there are also potential disadvantages, which include lack of anonymity and possible problems of tracing people. *For example, Clients are interested in following the mood of a small group of patients who have received a certain type of treatment. They expect that those who are high scorers on the mood questionnaire will remain high scorers throughout the study.*

Experimental and quasi-experimental approach

In this design, the group to be surveyed is divided into two or more smaller groups with the aim of doing some experimental or quasi-experimental study. An experimental study is one where a variable is manipulated or varied, and there are control groups within a randomized design; a quasi-experimental study is one where a variable is manipulated but there is no control group or the design is not fully randomized. Full experimental studies are usually better than quasi-experimental designs because stronger conclusions such as causality may be made. The classic way of designing such studies is to examine the effects of a variable of interest on one group (the experimental group), while not introducing the effect on a second group (i.e. the control group).

For example, we might be interested in determining whether patients responded positively to particular type of occupational therapy. One group of patients (the experimental group) could be assigned to the occupational therapy classes while another (the control group) might receive no occupational therapy. There might even be a third group (the placebo group), which is given a similar but meaningless type of occupational therapy that could be expected to be ineffective. After a set period of time, the difference in performance between start of therapy and finish of therapy could be measured by means of a questionnaire. This difference should be significantly larger and more positive than that of the control groups.

A Researcher may also be interested in determining the effect of music and lighting on staff productivity within operating theatres. It would be relatively easy to set up various different experimental conditions in which lighting and music were varied and administer a questionnaire afterwards on staff preferences.

In practice, such designs are rare within the health professions (except in the cases of clinical trials or similar) because it is generally poor practice from an ethical perspective to treat groups of people differently over a period of time simply for the purposes of data collection. For example, it seems unethical to subject patients to loud music when being operated upon! In the case of clinical trials, the ethical perspective is usually investigated very thoroughly prior to the study being approved.

Often there are also practical problems that also make experimental work with questionnaires and surveys difficult to undertake within the health professions. *For example, the Client is interested in determining whether patient care would be adversely affected by closing a certain ward at the weekend. It is unlikely that patients would be split into two groups (one group sent home at weekends and the other remaining at the ward) simply for the purposes of the survey, because of ethical and practical problems. On the other hand if this situation was already in operation then it is likely that the survey could be administered to the two groups. Note that this would then be a quasi-experimental design because subjects were not randomly assigned by the Researcher to one of the two groups.*

The different kinds of experimental design (such as, for example, controlling for patients' expectations and beliefs by means of placebo designs) are really beyond the scope of this text and unnecessary strictly from the perspective of questionnaire and survey design, so see De Vaus (1991), Oppenheim (1992), and Polit and Hungler (1991) for a fuller discussion on experimental design.

If it is too expensive, too difficult or unethical to set up a field experiment then it might be possible to conduct the study as a 'simulation' within a laboratory. For example, a Researcher would be unlikely to inflict wounds on individuals prior to determining staff treatment preferences by means of a questionnaire! The chances are that the Researcher would define several scenarios (or vignettes), or perhaps videotape some faked injuries, and then ask staff to complete the questionnaire based on these samples. These designs may not be 100% realistic to the staff, but they may be as realistic as it is possible to achieve given the practical and ethical limitations involved in setting up the study. Such designs also have the advantage that simulations can be relatively easy to contrive and administer to a schedule that is convenient to both the experimenter and the people being tested.

Summary

The design of the survey or questionnaire is as important as any other factor in the study. The Researcher must ensure that the survey design is appropriate for the kind of study that is required. There are two main types of simple survey design: (a) cross-sectional and (b) longitudinal.

In general, most surveys or questionnaire designs will be cross-sectional or longitudinal, but with multiple groups so that the design falls somewhere between the simple descriptive approach and the strict experimental design which is virtually impossible to achieve. These quasi-experimental designs will often be the best compromise that achieves the objectives of the survey while keeping the time, commitment and ethical implications to a reasonable level. One exception to this rule is clinical testing, in which it is important that far stricter experimental designs are followed. Here there are often one or more control groups.

It is important to note the practical and ethical implications of using multiple groups when conducting a survey within the health professions. To do something in one way to one group of subjects and in another way to another group of subjects may be ethically doubtful since by definition one group must be receiving worse treatment than the other. Unless there is good reason to perform the study, such designs may not pass ethical scrutiny – especially when conducted solely for the purposes of data collection. Occasionally there will be opportunities to collect data from multiple groups that have already been classified (such as patients who have already undergone different treatments, perhaps because of seeing different doctors). Although such quasi-experimental designs are less strong than full experimental designs, it is often possible to draw reasonable conclusions from these designs. Another possibility is to design a simulation of the experimental conditions.

Chapter 6
Choosing between postal and interview surveys

Introduction

When deciding upon survey method, the essential choice confronting the Researcher is to decide between postal surveys, interview surveys and computer administered surveys. Interview surveys can be direct (face-to-face) or indirect (telephone or videolink).

In terms of best practice, the Researcher needs to choose the administration method best suited for the survey or questionnaire that is to be used. You will notice in this chapter that the choice is not easy and will vary from situation to situation.

Postal surveys

Here Respondents receive the survey or questionnaire through the internal mail or through the post. Increasingly, the internet will also be used for this type of survey. When conducting a postal survey, the Researcher should prepare the mailing of the survey along the following lines:

(a) Include an initial letter (see Box 7) outlining the objective of the survey. The style of this letter can have a major effect on response rate. Include in the letter:
– official letterhead
– date of mailing
– name and address of the Researchers
– statement of purpose

- statement of how the person was selected
- an assurance of confidentiality if appropriate
- a statement of what will be done with the results
(c) Offer to send a summary of the results (*and subsequently do it!*).
(d) Keep the questionnaire short and simple. If personal questions have to be asked, explain why.
(e) Consider offering incentives, such as entry into a prize draw or book tokens.
(f) Be prepared to follow up or send reminders at set periods after the mailing.
(g) Be aware that the use of surveys and concern for ethical issues are interconnected. Surveys are conducted to obtain information, but the individual has a right to privacy.
(h) Completion and return mechanisms.

Another good rule is for Researchers to mail the survey on a Tuesday so that it reaches Respondents on a Thursday. This gives Respondents a chance to complete the survey at the weekend. Surveys should never be sent out in December or just before official holidays.

To achieve a good response, the Researcher should be prepared to remind people who have not returned the survey within a short time (1 to 2 weeks is usually appropriate). A second and even a third attempt to recover completed surveys should be made if there are sufficient funds, and if there are no problems with anonymity guarantees. The Researcher will need to have some method of matching returned questionnaires to the Respondents so that they can be contacted. This can raise issues of confidentiality if the survey is anonymous. It is better for the Researcher to impress on the Respondents the importance and urgency of the project than to use threats.

Ways to improve the response rate of mail questionnaires

Nachmias and Nachmias (1981) reviewed the best strategies for ensuring the optimal response rate for survey and questionnaire completion. Response rate can be increased by:

(a) Recognition of sponsors
   The right kind of sponsor (such as a well-known person, charity, religious group, etc.) can motivate Respondents to complete a

Box 7

Example cover letter

                              Department of Music Therapy
                              University Hospital of Beluga
                              Beluga
                              Onduras

                              Tel: (056) 945 234

Jane Eyres
235A Barley Road
Beluga
Onduras

[Date here]

Dear Jane Eyres,

Re: The effect of music therapy on your mental wellbeing

It is very important for us to determine the relative success of different types of therapy so that we provide the best quality care for our patients.

As someone who has recently attended our music therapy clinic here in the Department of Music Therapy at the University Hospital of Beluga, we are interested in your views of the therapy and in determining how well you feel now.

This is a new type of therapy and consequently we do not have a large number of people to survey. Together with our need to get a representative sample of patients, it is therefore of great importance to us that you complete the questionnaire and return it in the stamp addressed envelope provided.

Your answers will be completely confidential and will be used as part of a statistical analysis. The code at the top of the first page is used simply to check whether we have received your completed

(contd)

> questionnaire. Your name will never be placed on the questionnaire.
>
> We know a lot of our patients take great interest in this type of survey. If you would like a summary of the results please return the enclosed address label with the questionnaire. Please do not put this information on the survey itself.
>
> For further information please feel free to call me on 056 945 758.
>
> Thank you for your assistance.
>
> Yours sincerely
>
> Danielle Dupont
> Project Director

survey or questionnaire, and therefore the Researcher should include details of sponsorship in the covering letter. Sponsorship would appear to have the effect of making the survey more legitimate. It is also good practice from an ethical perspective to ensure that Respondents are fully informed of the identity of the sponsors.

(b) Inducement

Researchers can employ several types of inducement to try and improve response rate. The first is to appeal to the goodwill of the Respondents, perhaps by saying that their help is urgently required. The second is to offer a reward or a prize for successful completion. Nachmias and Nachmias find problems with this approach, however, because it seems as though some Respondents regard the usually nominal sum on offer as derisory and are therefore put off from completing the questionnaire. Usually a nominal reward is seen as no more than a symbolic gesture. The third method, which may be the best of all, is to appeal to Respondents' altruistic sentiments – perhaps by convincing them that the study is of great significance. All this can be expressed in the covering letter.

(c) Questionnaire format

Time spent on design and presentation of a survey is likely to pay dividends by increasing the response rate. Make the cover aesthetically pleasing, have a title that is interesting, make the pages of the questionnaire attractive to look at, and use an appropriate font and font size. It seems as though colour of survey has little effect. The length of a survey seems to affect the response rate – basically the shorter the questionnaire, the better the response rate. One can also set out the questionnaire economically so that a long questionnaire looks shorter.

(d) Cover letter

The cover letter is of great importance in convincing Respondents to complete and return the survey. The letter should therefore identify the survey sponsor, explain the purpose and significance of the study and assure anonymity (if it is on offer). It seems that a semi-personal style of letter can generate a slightly higher response rate than a formal letter.

(e) Include a stamped, self-addressed envelope (when needed)

It is unreasonable to expect Respondents to pay for the return of the survey or to address their own envelope for return of the questionnaire. According to Nachmias and Nachmias the response rate is better with stamps than with a business-reply envelope.

(f) Selection of respondents

Apart from the obvious proviso that the sample to be used in a study depends primarily upon the nature of the study, and thus there is very little that can be done about improving response rate by careful selection of Respondents, it seems as though certain types of Respondents are more likely to respond than others. Questionnaires specifically designed for certain groups are more likely to get higher response rates from those groups than from others because these Respondents are more likely to be able to identify with the goals of the project. In addition education level, likely level of interest and familiarity with the research project, and whether the respondents are professional or not may also affect the response rate.

(g) Follow-up

Follow-up is the most effective way of increasing the response rate. One common method is to send a reminder postcard (or similar) about one week after the questionnaire or survey has been sent out. About four weeks after the first mailing, the first replacement questionnaire can be sent and about seven weeks later the second replacement questionnaire can be sent. By using this method, the response rate in one study increased from 24% to 72%.

One problem with follow-up is anonymity, since this can no longer be assured if questionnaires are sent out only to those who have not replied. A way to get round this problem is to assure confidentiality of replies as opposed to anonymity. Another possible limitation to this method is that the quality of reply is likely to decrease as more reminders are sent out. Thus it may be that replacement questionnaires are more likely to be incomplete or defaced than the original questionnaires.

What is a suitable response rate?

There is no universal acceptable response rate since it depends upon so many other factors. The truth of the matter is that many mail questionnaires do not obtain return rates greater than 50% and this can be a problem because it may be that non-respondents are different in some important way to Respondents. Generally, a response rate of less than 35% might be considered unacceptable. For example, it seems that better-educated people from professional classes are more likely to be over-represented among Respondents, whereas others are likely to be less well represented. This problem can limit generalizability from a sample to an entire population.

It may also be that so many surveys and questionnaires are being sent out these days that potential Respondents feel over-burdened with them. Thus the overall response rate to surveys and questionnaires may be declining despite improved methods for increasing response rates.

Rea and Parker (1992) present minimum sample sizes for selected populations, and an adapted table of their results is shown in Table 2. This table represents a valuable rule of thumb but is certainly not completely infallible. After a certain point, it can be seen that the minimum sample size does not increase in proportion to the population size. For example, the minimum sample size to sample a population of 100,000 is not much bigger than that needed to sample a population of 10,000.

Henry (1990) builds on this work and presents a useful formula to adjust minimum sample size needed to take into account those unavailable to complete the survey and likely numbers of non-respondents.

The formula is:

N = O/P × R

where N = Adjusted minimum sample size, O = Minimum sample size, P = Proportion of available or eligible respondents, R = Response rate that can be expected. Imagine that a health manager wants to survey a hospital with 500 employees. Our figure suggests that a minimum sample of 218 is required, which needs to be adjusted upwards if only 70% of a sample can be considered to be available and the response rate is 75%:

N = 218/.70 × .75 = 415

The conclusion therefore would be that 415 of the 500 employees would need to be surveyed in order to obtain the minimum necessary sample size based on the assumptions and needs that have been stated. For different levels of confidence and different margins of error, see Rea and Parker (1992).

Practically, Clients are likely to want more than the minimum sample size surveyed as they may believe that the size simply would not be credible to a statistically unsophisticated audience. Moreover, sampling can increase mistrust and rivalry between members of the population being surveyed as they may typically wonder why some staff were included while others were excluded. A wise Researcher will note that human nature seems to conclude that inclusion or exclusion by chance is a highly improbable explanation, whereas conspiracy is a highly favoured explanation!

See Rea and Parker (1992) for a more detailed picture. Also note that response rate and availability are two other factors that will also need to be taken into account.

Types of interview survey

Interviews can be regarded as a social exchange between Interviewer and respondents, in which the Interviewer asks questions that the respondent answers. The most usual type of survey interview follows a structured schedule in which the questions, wording and the order of the questions is fixed. Thus every respondent is presented with a standardized interview. This approach is followed to ensure that

Table 2. Minimum sample sizes for selected small populations

Population size	95% confidence with 5% margin of error
< 200	Sample whole population
500	218
1,000	278
2,000	323
5,000	357
10,000	370
100,000	383

interview differences between respondents are not responsible for differences in the way questions are asked.

This kind of standardization is only possible if:

(a) Respondents have a common vocabulary
(b) Questions can be phrased so that they have the same meaning to all respondents
(c) All other components of the interview are the same for each Respondent (same interview manner, etc.).

An alternative type of interview is the non-structured interview in which no specific questions have been decided on beforehand and no standardized sequence of questions is used. The Interviewer has freedom to probe and the respondent is free to describe whatever is significant.

In some ways the structured interview and the non-structured interviews (see Box 8) are at the opposite ends of a continuum and many types of interview will fall in between. For example, one type of interview might structure the general format by defining all the general topics to be covered, but then allow the Interviewer and Respondent considerable freedom over how each of these general topics is to be covered. This allows the Interviewer to explore details, such as individual feelings about something, that would not be possible within a structured environment. Interviewers must be highly skilled, knowledgeable about the situation, and alert and sensitive to be successful at this type of interview.

Box 8

Example of different types of interview

Just as questions or items in pencil and paper surveys can have a closed or open format (see Chapter 9), interviews can also be structured or unstructured. By 'structured' we mean that the questions have been identified and agreed upon earlier. Thus the Interviewer's job involves reading out the questions and perhaps also recording the answers. On the other hand, the unstructured interview has not been previously planned and thus the Interviewer's questions are less well thought out but have the advantage of being able to zero in on the issues that are identified within the interview.

Structured interview

Within a structured interview, the Interviewer might say to the Respondents: 'We are interested in your ideas about the causes of heroin addiction and are not interested in your views about whether you yourself are an addict. There follows a list of some of the ways in which heroin addiction may be caused and we would like you to state your level of agreement to the following questions ...

(1) Their parents spent little time with them and rarely praised them
(2) They have failed to reach culturally desired goals
(3) They feel alienated from their society
(4) They cannot cope with their financial problems
(5) They have a lack of social and moral standards
(6) They have genetically inherited heroin addiction from their parents etc.

(adapted from a questionnaire by Furnham & Thompson, 1996)

Non-structured interview

Instructions to the Interviewer: Your task is to discover what Respondents believe to be the causes of heroin addiction. Be sure to mention at the start that we are not interested in whether they are addicts themselves but that you are simply interested in their views. Cover as many possible causes that the Respondent can think of and be alert to explore these different causes in depth.

Some of the differences between these types of interviews include:

1. Structured interviews are hard to design but easy to score and interpret
2. Non-structured interviews are easy to design but hard to interpret
3. Inexperienced Researchers tend to prefer non-structured interview designs because the planning is easy and they have not yet thought of the scoring problems!
4. Non-structured interviews are good when exploring an issue, as for example, when using focus groups to define items for later use in a structured interview.

Computer administered surveys

Computer administered surveys are likely to become increasingly popular. As more software becomes available, more people have access to computers, computers become networked and the internet becomes more widely used as a means of communication, it seems likely that the computer will become the survey administration method of choice.

The following points are useful to note:

(a) Respondents do not need to have much knowledge of computers to operate most computer administered questionnaires as they generally 'run themselves' and contain the operating instructions.
(b) Usually the questions are presented on the screen one at a time and the Respondent cannot go back more than one question. This has an advantage over a pencil and paper version of the questionnaire in that it concentrates the mind of the Respondent on each individual question and Respondents cannot keep going back and changing their answers. Usually, therefore, completion time is shorter by computer than by pencil and paper.
(c) Quality of presentation is much better with computers and branching questions are very easily handled within a computer program. Respondents usually also feel that this is a better way of answering questions than by simple pencil and paper format.
(d) Another advantage of computer administered surveys is that the Respondent does the data entry – saving time and improving accuracy.

(e) A further advantage is that computers can prevent Respondents from missing questions so often datasets are more complete than with pencil and paper formats.
(f) Sometimes the survey is sent out on a disk, completed by the Respondent and then returned. Quality control is essential that disks are not sent out with errors or with viruses. Care must also be taken when receiving the disks back since the Respondents may have unwittingly deleted or corrupted files or even copied viruses onto the disks.
(g) Networked computers, e-mail of the questions and answers, or use of the internet make it possible to distribute the questionnaire and receive the answers without having to send out the survey on a disk. It is via these methods that surveys will increasingly be conducted.

Do not use computer administered surveys when:

(a) Respondents do not have access to a computer
(b) The reliability of the hardware is poor
(c) Respondents have a wide range of different types of hardware and operating systems
(d) Respondents feel that this survey method would be intimidating
(e) The cost of the purchase of all this equipment is prohibitive
(f) The survey team is not competent in the use of the hardware and software required for successful implementation of the project.

Interview surveys

Pencil and paper surveys and computer administered surveys are normally 'posted' (either through the mail or electronically) to the individual. The usual alternative to posting is the interview survey, of which there are two types: **Direct** (face-to-face) and **indirect** (telephone, videolink).

Face-to-face surveys involve an Interviewer interviewing the Respondents when they are both in the same room. Telephone surveys and videolinks involve interviewing indirectly. Computer videolinks are an increasingly attractive alternative where the facilities exist.

When choosing between them, the following advantages of indirect methods over direct interviewing methods should be examined:

(a) Cost efficiency. Telephone surveys are much cheaper than face-to-face interviews, costing perhaps 200-400% less overall.
(b) Sampling efficiency. Telephone surveys *can* provide the Researcher with opportunities to collect relatively unbiased data. For example, it is possible to ask the person who answers the phone if he or she meets the sample requirements. If not, then it is possible to ask if there is another person in the household who meets the sample requirements, and to request an interview with them.
(c) Speed. Telephone surveys can be quick, even allowing for call-back to or from the Respondents.
(d) Telephone surveys can be less biased in terms of Interviewer bias than face-to-face interviews, especially in terms of gender, race or class biases.

Some of the major disadvantages of telephone surveys are:

(a) Telephone surveys must be brief and the range of possible answers to each question should be kept short because Respondents find the process tiresome. However once the interview has started people rarely hang up, so it is possible to continue for longer periods when necessary (even up to 30 minutes).
(b) The potential for unbiased sampling is large, even if there are ways to avoid this. Some of the problems to be overcome are:
  (i) Unlisted phone numbers or samples of the population that have few telephones. There tends to be a greater proportion of low-income city people with unlisted telephone numbers compared with richer people who live in the suburbs or country. Equally, some staff in the health professions will be easier to contact than others using the telephone. Random dialling can overcome the problems of unlisted telephones but not the problem of contacting staff who are difficult to reach on the telephone.
  (ii) People change their extension numbers or telephone numbers between updates of official telephone directories. Again random dialling can help solve these problems.
  (iii) People who answer the telephone at work (e.g. receptionists, secretarial staff) may not be the ones the Researcher is hoping to talk to.
  (iv) The phone might not be answered.
  (v) If answer phones are switched on only a message may reply.
  (vi) The telephone may be busy.

(vii) Different types of people are able to answer the phone at different times of day (because they work shifts, for example). Also people at work are unlikely to be surveyed by telephone calls during working hours to home numbers and people out of work are unlikely to be surveyed by calls to businesses.
(viii) Lists of numbers are often used in telephone surveys. These lists are usually out of date and/or do not cover the whole population. As such, some sections of the population in question may well be systematically under-represented.
(ix) People cannot remember a whole list of alternative response options with a telephone interview, whereas they can refer back to them with written survey formats.

See Lavrakas (1987) for more information about telephone surveys.

Principles of interviewing

The alternative to pencil and paper or computerized presentation of the survey is to interview the Respondents. Clearly, the interview as a general method for collecting information justifies a book in itself. Here is a very basic summary of the principles:

(a) Establish initial rapport with the Respondents
   Interviewers should:
   – Introduce themselves to the Respondents
   – Stimulate interest in the subject
   – Tell the Respondents how they were chosen
   – Set the Respondents at ease.
(b) Follow the interview guidelines
   Interviewers should:
   – Be informal and relaxed yet follow the structure and interview questions exactly as originally planned
   – Be prepared to repeat or clarify questions that the Respondent claims to misunderstand. Generally, however, this should not involve rewording the question.
(c) Probe
   Interviewers should:
   – Try to get Respondents to elaborate or clarify their answers, for example, by repeating elements of the Respondent's answer to try

to obtain more information but without including a direct or specific question

For example
>   RESPONDENT: *I first experienced symptoms of schizophrenia at about the age of 25.*
>   INTERVIEWER: *What kind of symptoms?*
>   RESPONDENT: *I felt really angry.*
>   INTERVIEWER: *Angry?*
>   RESPONDENT: *Yes. It seemed as though people were plotting against me.*
>   INTERVIEWER: *People. Anyone in particular?*
>   RESPONDENT: *My colleagues at work.*
>   INTERVIEWER: *Tell me more about this ...*

– Or be very specific in asking questions and then probe for further information

For example:
>   *An Interviewer is interested in obtaining information about the frequency, duration and intensity of headaches ...*
>   *How often do headaches currently occur?*
>   *How many have there been in the last month?*
>   *What about during the last week – how many headaches have you had?*
>   *Is that the typical pattern at present? How long has that been the case?*
>   *Has there been a noticeable change in the frequency of headaches, e.g. are they increasing, decreasing or just remaining the same?*
>   *How long do your headaches typically last?*
>   *What is the longest one you can remember?*
>   *What is the shortest?*
>   *Has the duration of your headaches altered over time?*
>   *How severe is the pain? Do your headaches vary in severity?*
>   *Can you describe it for me?*
>   *Can you remember the worst headache that you have ever had?*
>   *What was it like?*

(adapted from Wilson, Spence & Kavangh, 1989)

Mix of interview and questionnaire

Sometimes it seems to make sense for an Interviewer to be present, yet the Respondents complete the questionnaire themselves. Wellings, Field, Johnson, Wadsworth and Bradshaw (1994) present an example of the instructions used concerning the national survey of sexual attitudes and lifestyles:

'The next set of questions which are in this booklet will probably be easier if you read and answer them yourself. Some questions may not apply to you at all, so it shouldn't take too long to do. When you have finished, put the booklet in the envelope and seal it. It is very important to the study that you answer honestly and accurately, so please take your time. If you need any help or explanations, do please ask. I will just be doing some paper work whilst you do the booklet.'

Training and supervising the Interviewers

The Researcher needs to be aware that the art of interviewing well comes from skill and practice. As such, the Researcher must be committed to good preparation (see Box 9), which involves selecting and training the Interviewers. Again, here are a few good pointers:

(a) Select Interviewers especially on their presentation, powers of expression, voice quality, manner and motivation.
(b) Immediate feedback during training can improve interview manner considerably. Videotaping practice interviews and playing them back immediately can be effective in training.
(c) Let recruits learn interviewing technique by accompanying and listening to experienced Interviewers.
(d) Random checks are necessary to ensure Interviewers are doing their jobs correctly.
(e) Set up a system that ensures the procedure runs smoothly. It may be necessary to appoint a coordinator to plan the schedules and to keep track of the whole operation. Make sure that the planning, training and monitoring of the Interviewers is budgeted for in the original plan as this is something that is often missed, yet is very expensive.

Box 9

Key points about preparing for an interview survey

The following points are crucial to producing successful interview surveys:

(1) Type of Interviewer: Interviewers should fit in with, and possibly have the same sort of background as, the Respondents. They should be articulate and speak clearly. Their own attitudes should not influence the results. They should be closely monitored.
(2) Training: Systematic and intensive training of Interviewers is needed.
(3) Conducting interviews: Respondents should be interviewed alone. The Interviewer should make a brief introductory statement, outlining the aims of the survey and emphasizing the importance of the interview and of the answers. Interviewers should follow all instructions previously given in training; questions must be asked in the same order as listed in the survey.
(4) Monitoring Interviewers: This can take the form of an informal telephone conversation once a week, or the submission of a formal written report each day. It may be necessary to spend time with the person during interviews.

The in-depth Interviewer should be adequately prepared to:

(a) Carefully explain the purpose of the interview to the Respondent.
(b) Take time to relax the Respondent before beginning the interview.
(c) Be relaxed towards the Respondent.
(d) Assure complete confidentiality only if it is truly being offered.
(e) Be neutral and non-judgemental.
(f) Stick strictly to the written questions in the survey and ensure that the responses are correctly coded.
(g) Be careful about interviewing at the subject's place of work because of the danger of interruptions or having to sit in unpleasant or noisy surroundings.

Computer assisted telephone interviews

Increasing use of telephone survey methods has led to attempts to automate the process by using computers to dial the number, ask the questions, branch to various questions depending upon answer, identify answers which are inappropriate for the question, and store answers ready for analysis. Sometimes the Respondent may be asked to enter the answer by pushing the buttons on the telephone handset. Such methods are efficient, standardized and facilitate precise sampling, but they are, of course, expensive, especially when compared with a pencil and paper version.

Choosing between survey methods

Postal and interview survey methods are widely used methods of administration. The Researcher should choose between them by making informed choices based on the following criteria:

(a) Interviews can be flexible (depending upon structure) and can be adapted as they progress, whereas questionnaires are fixed and cannot be changed once sent out.
(b) Interviews can often collect key, contextual and unique information faster than posted questionnaires, but posted questionnaires can often collect information from large numbers of people faster.
(c) With interviews it is possible to ask for further explanations and provide more information about the Respondent's reactions. Because of this, complex and open-ended questions are best asked in an interview.
(d) Interviews can be useful if the Researcher is worried about the reading ability of the Respondents (this may be because of poor reading skills or because the survey is not written in the Respondents' first language).
(e) Respondents are more likely to be happy with one type of method than another. Although preference can be unpredictable, many Respondents will prefer the interview method because they feel that they can explain themselves better.
(f) Interviews entail a much greater financial burden than postal surveys because of the greater number of person-hours that are involved in doing interviewing, the costs of finding and training the Interviewers (essential!) and the costs of arranging the interviews.

(g) Gaining access to people to perform an interview can be difficult especially when they have dogs, are afraid to answer the door, etc. Moreover there can be dangers involved in night-time travel and working alone with strangers
(h) Postal surveys are more discreet than interviews as the survey form can be returned anonymously. With interviews, anonymity is more difficult to obtain, or – just as importantly – be seen to be obtained.
(i) Postal surveys are convenient for both the Researcher and the Respondents whereas interviews require a planned timetable. Having a timetable improves the chance of collecting information from a larger proportion of selected Respondents, which can reduce sampling bias.
(j) Interviewers can also introduce bias because Respondents may react differently to different interview styles and may note down answers in a biased manner.
(k) In general postal surveys have a low response rate, although there are methods for improving the response rate.
(l) It is much more difficult than in an interview or telephone survey to control who completes a questionnaire, as people may not pass it on to the appropriate person.
(m) Mail questionnaires and telephone surveys must be relatively quick whereas interviews can be longer. De Vaus (1991) adds a caveat that is worthwhile noting, however: the more specialized the population and the more relevant the topic, the longer the questionnaire can be. Sometimes it appears that short questionnaires can be seen as too trivial to waste time on.
(n) Many items remain unanswered with mail questionnaires whereas with interviews the Interviewer can often ensure questions are not missed.
(o) When the Respondent needs to be guided through the questionnaire (for example, the Respondent may only have to answer a subset of the questions) then the interview or telephone format is best since mail questionnaires tend to look overly long.

The Researcher should consider using the internet or intranet (an internet local to a specific organization) to administer a pencil and paper questionnaire. The advantages of computerized administration are that once the software has been written the costs of sending out the questionnaire and receiving the incoming data are low. If the survey is properly set up, the answers are also received in an electronic form ready for statistical analysis by computer. Moreover, the use of such a medium may increase response rate since Respondents will find the use of modern techniques interesting and stimulating.

There are many examples of questionnaires on the internet, covering a diverse range of interest.

Summary

The Researcher needs to choose between postal surveys and interview surveys. De Vaus (1991) summarizes the position as follows:

> 'if any broad conclusions were to be drawn about how to administer questionnaires it would be that face-to-face surveys are normally better at obtaining representative samples and produce the fewest constraints in terms of questionnaire construction and question design, with mail questionnaires the least satisfactory in these respects. But the reverse is true as far as the quality of answers is concerned: mail questionnaires are likely to be the best in this regard while face-to-face interviews encounter more problems than either mail or telephone methods. In general, face-to-face interviews are the least satisfactory when it comes to the practicalities of administration while mail and telephone methods have considerable, though different, advantages. In the end it is impossible to decide which method is best: the relative strengths and weaknesses vary according to the characteristics of the survey.' (pp. 112–13).

The words are simple but the message is complex – basically the Researcher should choose the survey method as a balance between the various factors that are relevant to the survey under consideration.

Chapter 7
Obtaining the right size and type of sample

Introduction

The most obvious way to discover information about a group of people is to collect that information from every single person in that group. This solution is fine with regard to small samples (say of less than 200). However, a problem emerges with larger groups in which the cost increases and the amount of time and energy involved becomes impractical in relation to the increase in accuracy.

The only sensible alternative is to collect the information from only some of the people in the group while ensuring that the information reflects the characteristics of the whole group. If this is done correctly then the information which is collected still has real meaning but the procedure is much cheaper, faster and easier than if the whole group had been surveyed. This is known as sampling, as opposed to a census in which information is collected about all the members of a particular group.

The understanding of a few key words will be useful when taking an overview of how to sample from a large group of individuals:

> **population** – all the members of a particular group
> **sample** – a subset of a population
> **representative sample** – a sample whose characteristics represent the population
> **biased sample** – a sample whose characteristics do not represent the population
> **sampling error** – the differences between the sample that is collected and the perfectly representative population
> **standard error** – the technique used to report the sampling error.

Once the survey has been designed, the Researcher needs to develop a very good idea of the group that will be sent the survey. The question arises whether to include every person in the group, or survey a portion only (i.e. to take a sample). The Researcher's decision depends on:

(a) how quickly the data are needed
(b) the type of survey
(c) the available resources (in terms of cost and time)
(d) the need for credibility (the more people who are surveyed, the higher the credibility).

Good survey design therefore requires that a representative sample is derived from the population or that the whole population is measured (if it is small enough). There are two broad types of sample: probability and non-probability. With a probability sample, each member of the population has an equal (or at the very least a known) probability of being selected. With a non-probability sample, some people have a greater (and unknown) chance than others of being selected.

Equal probability sampling

In this technique all participants have an equal probability of being selected from the main group. The resulting sample is required to be fully representative, essentially a miniature version, of the main group. Hence the sample is said to be representative. Several methods are available:

(a) **Simple random sampling:** A subset of Respondents is chosen at random from the group. The Researcher should use random number generators (e.g. simple tables, computer programs, specialized electronic equipment) to generate the list and should report the method used. The main advantages of this method are that it is very simple, understandable and easy to perform. This is the method that less experienced Researchers will tend to follow without understanding the disadvantages, which are that it:
(i) tends to produce greater errors in the results unless the sample is truly representative of the population. *For example, at any one*

time, sections of the health professions population will be difficult to contact at short notice by mail or telephone because they may be in transit, in a difficult-to-contact geographical location, or because records showing their location are wrong.

(ii) cannot easily be used when it is required to differentiate between subgroups (e.g. between male and female Respondents of different rank). *For example, the health professions are interested in determining job satisfaction of their personnel within a given organization. It would be possible to administer randomly a questionnaire so that a representative sample was obtained. Whilst this method would probably collect representative proportions of men and women of different seniority, it is unlikely that the average job satisfaction of, for example, male physiotherapists, could be calculated very accurately because there would only be a very small number within the representative sample.*

(b) Stratified random sampling: This method deals directly with the problem of subgroups. The population is first divided into appropriate meaningful subgroups (e.g. male medical staff; female medical staff; male administrators; female administrators) and then a given number of Respondents is selected randomly from each group. The process requires more effort, and will usually involve a larger sample size to give statistically meaningful results. As a general rule, which should not be applied too literally because it is very dependent upon the situation, the Researcher should aim for at least 30 people in each subgroup although quite often more would be desirable (more than 100 if possible). If necessary, overall mean scores can be calculated by weighting the subgroup means in relation to the true population proportions of the subgroups.

Non-probability sampling

Non-probability sampling is generally easier to perform, but may lead to greater error in the results of the survey. The method involves some degree of selection, either by accident or by design; hence participants do not have an equal chance of being selected.

(a) Opportunistic sampling: In this technique, the sample is obtained in a completely unsystematic way (e.g. the first 50 individuals leaving the doctors' canteen could be questioned about their views on a certain subject). The method tends to give biased results and is unconvincing.

(b) **Systematic sampling:** A list of participants is drawn up, and every nth name is selected for the survey. For example, if there were 1,000 names on the list and 200 were required, every fifth individual would be selected. A danger is that the list itself may contain a particular pattern arising from the way it was compiled, and this could then introduce bias into the survey. Again this method is not recommended.

(c) **Purposive sampling:** The sample is selected from groups who are known to have special qualifications. The latter may be based on knowledge, experience, or the holding of 'typical' views. Inaccuracy occurs because the Researcher may have grouped the participants in an inappropriate manner. Therefore, this technique can only be defended if the Researcher can justify the choices that have been made.

Finding the sample

Having decided on the sampling method, the Researcher has to locate the chosen Respondents and communicate with them. This may involve obtaining personnel lists from departments within the health professions. In many circumstances, permission should be sought before this type of information can be requested. It is not good practice to obtain the information through unofficial channels since this can leave the Researcher in a very exposed position if things go wrong.

Summary

The Researcher should:

(a) Choose a sampling method that ensures the sample used in the survey is representative of the population being studied
(b) Use a sampling method that represents a reasonably efficient use of resources, time and effort
(c) Ensure that the sample can be contacted through official channels.

Part 3:
Survey and questionnaire formats

Chapter 8
Generating the items

Introduction

The Researcher is now ready to add detail to the emerging survey or questionnaire by generating the items that will be used as a first draft prior to polishing for use in the trial run and the actual survey itself.

Developing the concepts to be used in the study

The creation of a survey begins with a set of observations and the development of a theory that explains these observations. This is the basis of good practice because it follows the scientific approach as described in Chapter 2. Once a Researcher has made a series of observations about a subject, the basic concepts underlying the survey or questionnaire need to be identified. The most important question is whether each observation is unique or whether it can be grouped with others. *For example, a Researcher may observe that a greater proportion of women seems to suffer from anorexia nervosa than men. Should gender be a single issue in a survey? It may be, for example, that gender (i.e. one's sex role in terms of femininity or masculinity) is of more consequence, or it could be that men and women have different body images, or it could be that women are exposed to greater media advertising about thinness. The main point is that the observation of a gender difference could be taken at face value as the basic concept of the observation or could be broken down into even more basic components of the subject area.*

The question of how a Researcher should know what general principles underlie a collection of observations is not simple to answer. Researchers have to be self-critical and questioning but, perhaps above all, they should be creative. However the development of theory is usually critical to the development of a survey or questionnaire since it puts all the observations into general principles that can be investigated or tested.

The importance of theory to the design of the survey or questionnaire must not lead to the theory becoming 'sacred' or 'untouchable'. The opposite is in fact true. A good Researcher will often set about looking for evidence that will disprove a theory as opposed to supporting it. *For example, if Researchers developed a theory that malaria was spread by only a certain type of mosquito, they could spend all their time testing this type of mosquito to see if it spread malaria. However, a single observation that a different type of mosquito was involved in the spread of malaria would disprove the hypothesis straight away and lead the Researchers to new and testable theories that they would then set about trying to disprove.*

Often 'flesh' is added to the 'bone' of the core concepts developed by the Researcher by means of in-depth interviews or focus groups and/or the design of a blueprint. The techniques described here basically involve getting experts to write about the subject in question, extracting the critical components of a particular problem and then putting structure into the items.

The in-depth pilot interview with subject experts

The Researcher's purpose in conducting the in-depth interview is to collect critical components that need to be included as items in the survey or questionnaire. Apart from this most important reason, in-depth interviews can help identify jargon used by the Respondents so that the survey is written in a meaningful way; promote good public relations because they create the impression of 'communal ownership'; serve to find out what is acceptable and unacceptable in terms of items and format to the Respondents; and finally serve to identify items and issues that should not be included in the survey. Taken together, the benefits of conducting in-depth pilot interviews and/or focus groups more than outweigh the costs and time involved in setting up the whole project.

The Interviewer conducts individual interviews with as many *representative* subject experts as possible within time, budget and availability constraints (perhaps optimally 30 or 40, but realistically more than 10). Sometimes when there are constraints group interviews will be conducted instead of individual interviews. The aim is to record (usually on tape but sometimes simply by pen and paper) detailed comments about the subject matter of the survey for later analysis.

For the purposes of information collection, the in-depth Interviewer:

(a) should be vague about the purpose of the interview (whenever possible) as spontaneous reactions are wanted.
(b) should be relaxed in the approach taken with the subject expert.
(c) should be neutral and non-judgemental during the interview but should be critical of what has been said when analysing the results, especially when asking people why they act or think as they do.
(d) should show authority but maintain a pleasant manner.
(e) must assure complete confidentiality.
(f) must ask the subject's permission to record the information either on audio or videotape.
(g) should avoid asking leading questions.
(h) should provide feedback to the interviewees to ensure that the recorded information is accurate.
(i) should be careful about interviewing at the subject's place of work because of the danger of interruptions or having to sit unpleasant or noisy surroundings.

One way of phrasing questions that extracts attitudes, values and beliefs relevant to a certain survey or questionnaire, and which is very effective at eliciting information, is by contrasting people known to the interviewees. *Taking the example of a questionnaire being designed to select high-performing midwives, the method progresses along the following lines. 'Imagine the best-performing midwife you have ever known. Now imagine the worst-performing midwife you have ever known. In what ways were they different? What was it that made the midwife such a good (poor) performer? How do experienced midwives differ from those recently recruited?*

A further way of extracting information of this sort is to ask experts about their working day. What do they do during the day? Why? What are the critical components of the job?

After the interview has been conducted, the Researcher and colleagues should listen to the tape and extract the key critical points from the interview. With regard to surveys that are designed to collect facts, it should be easy enough to formulate the items directly from this point. However, for surveys that are designed to collect opinions, the process is more difficult and requires structuring, possibly using the process described in the section entitled 'Finding the sample' in Chapter 7.

Focus groups

The focus group is far from new, dating from as far back as the Second World War, when people were asked to discuss openly their reaction to a radio programme after rating it. Since then, focus groups have been used primarily to discover attitudes and motivation for the purpose of initial survey design or to represent the views of particular groups and communities without the need to undertake a survey. Our view is that focus groups can be useful in the design of a survey or questionnaire but that they can never do the job of a survey or questionnaire because of the very small sample and the way that the data are collected.

A typical focus group consists of a moderator questioning and listening to a group of individuals discussing a particular topic or reacting to a particular product. It usually lasts for one to two hours and is ideally conducted in a 'comfortable setting'. This 'sensitive, qualitative' technique is akin to a think-tank situation. Sessions can take on a life of their own, often revealing myriad unexpected outcomes. The moderator's tasks are to encourage and challenge, as well as manage, disruption, diversion and other problem dynamics. Focus groups should ideally allow the moderator sufficient time and an appropriate setting to probe for, and draw out, important attitudes, perceptions, prejudices and opinions. Participant responses may be recorded by an observer/note-taker or a tape recorder, the former being easier to use because of the difficulty of knowing what was going on when listening to the tape.

The group is typically composed of between six and 10 individuals who have something in common. The ideal is to carry on running these groups until no novel information arises. This is, of course, potentially time wasting and enormously expensive, because it is never clear when some new, worthwhile data may arise. There is also no consensus on how to 'play the group' – to make sure everyone has equal time to speak, to encourage or discourage disagreement, to deal with dominant, distracting or dreary participants. In short, there are no clear guidelines of best practice, which is not good news for the person commissioning the focus group report.

The central idea of the focus group is to hear the language and ideas of ordinary people, to see how 'amateurs' represent and debate on topical issues. For some Researchers, the process is as important as the content – how people who do not know each other negotiate, discuss and attempt to persuade. The product of focus groups is usually a report, and these differ enormously in length, style and depth. They are characterized by having many quotes and by the essentially wry, perceptive interpretations of the observer on what, how and why ideas were generated.

Some Researchers like to call back groups over time, perhaps meeting weekly for a couple of months (like a company board or committee). Most, however, are 'one-off' experiences. The question of how to recruit and motivate participants is also unclear, but crucially important. Who volunteers for a focus group and do they have different opinions from non-volunteers? Some groups turn into self-help groups, others into political debating chambers and still others into social occasions with free coffee and biscuits and a present to take home. Perhaps most important of all is the role of the report-writer, if that is not the mediator. The long, jumbled, indeed often garbled, notes or recordings need to be 'written up' into a report. This, of necessity, involves interpretation, highlighting and selecting core themes, major points of dissension and even implicit and badly articulated ideas. Precisely how this is done and how reliable is the interpretation is never clear.

The limitations of this technique are very clear:

1. It is difficult to make generalizations from these small, deliberately unrepresentative samples and results may be unreliable: run two groups and you will get quite different results. Have different moderators and interpreters for the same group and you will also have two very different reports on which to base the survey design. In short, the results are not replicable. And something that is unreliable can, by definition, rarely be valid; it seems focus groups do not measure what they say they are measuring.
2. Public ideas are problematic, pluralistic, conflicting, diverse and contradictory. The focus group stresses (indeed, often glorifies) this and yields results that are no help to the decision maker. Rather than clarifying the situation, focus group reports tend to

make it worse. In a sense, the reports rejoice in indecisiveness and plurality, rather than a consensus – whether it is there or not.
3. Even the most skilful moderator cannot overcome the fundamental problem of groups making decisions, because:
   (a) people have evaluation apprehension – some self-censor, being scared to look foolish, and will never say in public forum (the very open focus group) what they really think.
   (b) social loafers will go along for the spectacle and the 'freebies' but contribute little, letting the garrulous speak for them. In this sense, the focus group reports are biased towards the eloquent and opinionated who might not speak for the group. In fact, some moderators go out of their way to choose the talkative, as they yield more material.
   (c) it is difficult to think about a problem seriously when some know-all is continually talking. That is, they allow little or no quiet time to think about the issue before giving one's opinions.
   (d) there are powerful conformity pressures to take sides and follow certain individuals or subgroups; in short to obey explicit and implicit upheld norms, giving a misleading idea of the spread of ideas in the group

A few years ago brainstorming groups were all the rage. The research on these groups showed, however, that compared to the pooled ideas of people working alone, brainstorming groups nearly always produced *fewer* and *lower quality* innovative ideas. Focus groups, being in many ways similar, share the same limitations.

Focus groups do have a certain fascination. They often yield great quotes, provoke powerful emotions and even cause people to come to blows. One can pretend that, as the mediator or interpreter, one has special trained insights, allowing one to speak for or interpret the otherwise tongue-tied or incoherent. This is a dangerous myth. If you want to know what people really think, or even, more importantly, how they are going to react, you need to interrogate a large representative sample in a situation of sufficient anonymity and confidentiality to understand the real values, motives and behaviour intentions. One needs to question their attitudes, behavioural intentions and past behaviours. Focus groups, it seems, are for the short-sighted. 'Hocus pocus' is defined in the dictionary as 'a pointless activity, or words often intended to obscure or deceive'. This is just what many focus groups turn out to be, no matter how well intentioned.

Structuring the contents of the questionnaire

The next step is for the Researcher to develop the survey items from the knowledge base that has been accumulated by means of the interview or focus group. One recommended way is to develop a grid structure in which content area is the horizontal axis of the table and items are the vertical axis (see Rust and Golombok, 1989). One further note is that this process is often conducted with subject experts, or evaluated by subject experts prior to producing the actual items used in the survey.

	Content areas			
	1	2	3	4
Items				
(a)				
(b)				
(c)				
(d)				
(e)				

Each content area should not have much of an overlap with other content areas. *For example, a survey designed to measure doctors' managerial qualities may have several different content areas called Autocracy, Charisma, Support, etc. Another example, a survey to measure the usefulness of a new type of syringe, may have content areas of: Ease of use, Safety, etc.*

The Researcher then selects items providing a broad and complete description of each content area. To continue with the second example, it may be decided that 'Ease of use' is a simple enough content area for there to be no need to split it up into components. However, it is also possible that it could be split into: (a) Easy to fill (b) Easy to inject, etc.

For attitude surveys in which Respondents will be asked to provide an opinion, a good rule is to use more than 10 items to cover each content area to help ensure reasonable internal reliability for each content area (but never use tautologies to achieve this goal). For objective surveys, in which Respondents will be asked to report a 'factual truth', the items in the survey will generally be much clearer and so rules are less important. *For example, a survey designed to measure staff priorities over the next five years may take the following form (note that this is a simplification). Three content areas are chosen and named:*

(a) Achievement and prestige
(b) Career progression
(c) Structured work

Once the content areas have been identified then items are selected to fit the content area:

	Content areas		
	1 Achievement and prestige	2 Career progression	3 Structured work
Items			
(a)	Feel like you are accomplishing something	Promotion on the basis of ability	Work under intelligent work policies
(b)	Be in a competitive situation	Advance at a rapid rate	Travelling
(c)	Work spouse can be proud of	Be given recognition for work well done	Definite work schedule
(d)	Prestige and social status	Achieve leadership in your field	Spend time with family

Together with the experts, the Researcher identifies items for the survey to fit each of these content areas. As shown above, the first four items associated with Achievement and prestige are:

(a) Feel like you are accomplishing something
(b) Be in a competitive situation
(c) Doing work spouse can be proud of
(d) Obtaining prestige and social status

It is possible then to produce a *first draft* of the items that will form the survey. At this stage, the Researcher should only produce a rough draft because writing the items is complex and will be fully covered later in the book. The first draft (containing the full range of items) may look something like this:

This survey sets out to determine staff priorities over the coming year. Please rate the importance of the following items:

1. Feel like you are accomplishing something
2. Obtain promotion on the basis of ability
3. Work under intelligent work policies
4. Be in a competitive situation
5. Advance at a rapid rate
6. Attend conventions
7. Do work spouse can be proud of
8. Be given recognition for work well done
9. Have a definite work schedule
10. Obtain prestige and social status
11. Achieve leadership in your field
12. Spend time with family

Tidying up the items and adding a rating scale such as:

5 = Extremely important for me to obtain
4 = Important for me to obtain
3 = Neither important nor unimportant
2 = Unimportant for me to obtain
1 = Extremely unimportant for me to obtain

will be covered at a later stage in the survey design (see Chapter 9). A more complete example is shown in Box 10.

Box 10

Topics to consider: How people overcome depression

As another example, here is a list of possible questionnaire items that describe ways in which people might overcome or cope with depression. (Each item could be rated with a five-point scale with bipolar categories of Strongly disagree vs Strongly agree.) Without research, such a list would be incomplete and therefore a whole research project could be flawed right from the start.

Overcoming depression depends upon:

(a) How hard a person tries.
(b) How much willpower (inner strength) a person has.
(c) How lucky a person is.
(d) Whether a person gets professional help.
(e) How much information a person has about the problem.
(f) A person's general ability to overcome problems.
(g) Whether the problem is a symptom of some other deep-rooted problem.
(h) Whether the person believes it is possible to eliminate the problem.
(i) How embarrassed the person feels about having the problem.
(j) How damaging the problem is to the person's feelings of self-worth or self-esteem.
(k) How much eliminating the problem would please others.
(l) How much a person stays away from situations that make the problem worse.
(m) How much a person understands about the underlying reasons for the problem.
(n) How much self-control the person has.
(o) Whether the person gets help from other people (friends and loved ones).
(p) How intelligent the person is.
(q) How much the person believes in God.
(r) How much the person stays away from others with similar problems.

Generating the items

> (s) Whether there is something wrong with the person's brain or nervous system.
> (t) Whether the person's mother and/or father have a similar problem
> (u) Whether the person seeks out trained medical/psychological help.
> (v) How much the person wants to get better.
> (w) Whether the person joins other self-help groups for this problem.
> (x) How much courage a person has to change his or her life style.
>
> These 24 items seem to be a succinct and balanced list of the kinds of ways in which people may overcome depression.

Using exploratory factor analysis to structure the questionnaire

It certainly is possible for Researchers in survey and questionnaire design to add structure to the survey without collecting data and performing an 'exploratory factor analysis'. In other words, Researchers can identify patterns in the questions and determine which questions seem to tap into the same underlying attitudes without performing complex statistical analyses. This will be a relief for many survey designers because factor analysis is a complex multivariate statistical procedure that will be too difficult for most inexperienced Researchers.

However, many experienced Researchers would prefer to use a statistical method of classifying items into content areas rather than relying on the subjective judgement methods described in the previous section. We describe the process of factor analysis in Chapter 11 and also refer the interested reader to Kline (1994), who provides a relatively easy guide to factor analysis.

Here we simply provide a basic list of the process of exploratory factor analysis and show an example in Box 11 of how items numbers might be reduced in this process.

1. Conduct a pilot study to gather data for use in the analysis (see Chapter 10)

2. Determine the number of factors to be extracted. The two most common methods are to use the scree slope methodology or the number of factors with eigenvalues greater than one.
3. Extract and rotate the factors to provide as simple a solution as possible. The most common rotation procedure is known as the varimax method.
4. Examine the items which are related to each of the factors and name the factors according to these items.

Box 11

Example of item selection methodology

1. Review of literature provides six items from scale.
2. Focus group provides interesting quotes from which five items are derived.
3. Pilot interview with five experts and five lay people derives nine items.
4. A first draft of the questionnaire is written.
5. Evaluation of draft by new group of experts and lay people who are asked to add and improve the items. This adds a further 10 items.
6. End up with 30 items.
7. Pilot the questionnaire and then use factor analysis to split the items into specific content areas or sections.
8. Draw up the final questionnaire.

Summary

When writing the first draft of the items, the Researcher needs to:

(a) know the subject area by conducting appropriate research
(b) develop the items (if they do not exist already) by means of interviews and focus groups
(c) construct items that express a component of the content area whilst not overlapping too much
(d) determine if the structure fits in with experts' opinions
(e) possibly collect data and perform exploratory factor analysis to determine the statistical structure of the survey or questionnaire
(f) be prepared to further tailor the items according to the results.

Chapter 9
Writing the survey

Introduction

The first task for the Researcher to consider when actually preparing to sit down and write the final draft of the survey items is to think about the general format of the survey. Basically, this requires the Researcher to make informed judgements about:

(a) length of survey
(b) order of questions in survey
(c) aesthetics and other concerns such as layout, use of logos, etc.

Once the general format has been decided upon, the Researcher can then fully develop the items. Choices of item type essentially revolve around choosing closed or open-ended questions. Closed questions can usually be answered by a simple yes/no assessment, ticking a checklist or providing a rating. Open-ended questions deal with the more complex concepts to which a closed question will not be able to provide a full response. Analysis of open questions is likely to be very difficult, especially since it includes the interpretation of another person's expressions and terms. It often involves a very lengthy process of defining categories that can be used to classify the answers to the open questions.

Length of survey

The length of a survey depends on the following factors:

(a) The number of content areas that are required and the number of items in each content area that are necessary to give credible data. A good rule is to have at least 10 items making up each content area in which an opinion is sought to ensure reasonable reliability (*but if only one or two items are appropriate without repetition or tautology, then use only one or two!*).
(b) Type of survey. Self-administered questionnaires contain fewer items and are generally limited to about 20 minutes; face-to-face interviews may contain many more items and may take longer. Telephone interviews should be short since the Respondent may get tired but, on the other hand, it may be possible to prolong the telephone interview since many Respondents are reluctant to 'hang up'.
(c) The amount of time Respondents have available and how much they are prepared to give.
(d) The resources available to the Researcher.

Order of questions in the survey

The Researcher should plan the survey to:

(a) Start with a straightforward introduction, personal details and then questions related to the objective (see Box 12 for an example set of first questions for an anonymous survey).
(b) place sensitive questions in the middle or near the end.
(c) end with the easy questions (as the Respondents may be getting tired).

Box 12

Example of a personal details section of an anonymous survey

This questionnaire concerns your personal attitudes and behaviour regarding the use of complementary (*alternative*) and *general* medicine. By complementary medicine we mean treatment such as acupuncture, homeopathy, herbalism and osteopathy. The questionnaire presents a number of statements representing aspects concerning health. You are asked to read each question carefully and we ask you to be honest in your responses. Most of the questions require you to give a response to the amount you agree, disagree, or the amount to which you do something. The higher the number, the more you agree or do what the question states. Most responses require you to tick or circle a number. *Your anonymity is assured and your help is appreciated.*

Personal details

1. Sex (circle):   Male   Female

2. Year of birth: 19___

3. Number of years of formal schooling: _____

4. Do you have a degree?   Yes   No

5. Marital status (circle): Single   Married   Widowed   Divorced   Cohabiting   Other

6. Number of children (circle): 0 1 2 3 4 5 6 7 More

7. Please describe your current occupation or your occupation when last employed. Be as explicit as you can (i.e. painter in an auto garage, sales manager in a clothing store, 6th grade science teacher, etc.).

8. To which income bracket do you belong (circle):

< £5,000   £5,001–8,000   £8,001–10,000   £10,001–15,000
£15,001–20,000   £20,001–30,001   £30,000+

Here we display some interesting personal details questions for an anonymous survey. Questions 1 to 3 represent fairly standard questions to which a straightforward reply could be expected. Question 4 has been carefully designed to collect simple information relevant to the study. To ask more in-depth questions about education would necessarily involve a more complex type of question with many response alternatives. Questions 5 and 6 are examples of questions in which we need to provide all response alternatives. Question 7 is

(contd)

> an open-ended question that allows complex information to be provided by the Respondent while keeping the actual question very simple. This does, however, mean that scoring of this question can be difficult. Question 8 asks people to circle their current income. Note the unequal size of the categories. This was probably done by the Researchers so that a reasonable number of Respondents would circle each of the possible options.

Then the Researcher should observe the following rules:

(a) Proceed in a logical order that makes sense while also following a natural sequence as far as possible.
(b) Deal with objective questions before subjective ones.
(c) Move from the most familiar items to the least familiar items.
(d) Avoid introducing personal bias.
(e) Maintain the Respondent's interest (e.g. avoid repetition in question content or format, think about using colours and interesting presentation methods, such as cartoons, diagrams, etc.).
(f) Randomize the order of items in particular sections if the Researcher does not want Respondents to become aware of the underlying scales (*for example, if asking questions about leadership qualities then randomize the items that belong to different facets of leadership*). However when it is more convenient to the Respondent to keep the items in order, then do so (*for example, when conducting a survey on religious affairs, ask all the items relating to the Chaplain, then the chapel, etc.*)
(g) Present closed questions before open questions.
(h) Do not use too much spacing – Respondents prefer to complete short questionnaires (or at least those that look short based on page length!).

Survey format: aesthetics and other concerns

The appearance of the survey is important. It should be clear and easy to read, and provide sufficient space for answers to be recorded while not being over-generous. The Researcher should place one question on one line, and not squeeze several questions together. The response format should leave sufficient space for the Respondent to make the appropriate remarks.

Branching questions may be used when asking about a topic that will not be relevant to everyone participating in the survey. *For example, a general attitude survey may address issues that are relevant to just one group of staff within the health professions, although all groups are sent the questionnaire. There may therefore be branching questions that direct female doctors, for example, to one section of the survey and male doctors to another.*

Nachmias and Nachmias (1981) describe several formats suitable for branching questions:

(a) Write directions next to each response category of the filter question (such as go to Question 33).
(b) Use arrows to direct the Respondent to the next appropriate question.
(c) Box each set of contingencies to set them apart from the more usual type of items in a survey or questionnaire.

The Researcher should also make sure the design of the survey is attractive – the survey is sent out to many Respondents, and from this pool there will always be those who are critical and negative. Good design and well-presented documentation will improve the chances of the survey's success.

Open-ended questions

A typical survey involving open-ended questions might be designed to determine how satisfied, or dissatisfied, customers are with a particular product or service. A standard approach is to ask Respondents to list at least one thing, but no more than three things, that they like best (or least) about the subject. Then the Researcher should proceed with the content analysis as follows:

(a) List all the answers given.
(b) Subdivide the answers into categories of closely related responses (probably with the aid of experts). Then check the categories, again using experts, and it will often be found that some categories may require splitting and others grouping together.
(c) Give a code number to each category.
(d) Tabulate the number of responses for each code.
(e) Analyse the participants' response pattern.

In general, open-ended questions are easy to plan but difficult to analyse and draw conclusions from. Problems arise from difficulty in producing exhaustive, non-overlapping categories and then applying the definitions of these categories in a consistent manner.

Best practice in survey design generally advises against the use of open-ended questions. Sometimes the use of open questions indicates that the Researcher has not put sufficient thought into the design stages of the survey – the open questions reflect a failure to research the area properly and to develop well thought-out scales that describe the important content areas of the topic. Having said this, it is also true that open questions can provide forthright and valuable insights into people's perceptions of the issues involved and to get a feel for the words and phrases that they use.

Closed questions

Closed questions are in the form of a statement or a question, followed by several boxes representing alternative choices. The following factors are important in constructing questions:

(a) Keep questions strictly relevant. A Researcher should be able to justify the inclusion of every question.
(b) Each question should show direct relevance to the central topic of the survey. Avoid introducing items that the Respondent will not readily associate with the survey.
(c) Use standard English and aim for short, clear, and precise sentences. Do not employ specialized technical terms or jargon; abbreviations are only acceptable if they are defined when first introduced or are well known to all Respondents. Avoid double negatives.
(d) Questions should be direct and to the point. Do not introduce abstract concepts.
(e) Beware of bias and unintentional offensiveness (especially with regard to race, disability, religion or sex differences).
(f) Responses to questions may be influenced by phrases or words used in the question (see Box 13). Moreover, the acceptability of the survey to the Respondents is very important and offensive questions can reflect badly on the survey designer. The Researcher needs to ensure that biases are not reflected in the phraseology chosen.

> **Box 13**
>
> ## Contradictory evidence from surveys: we want to pay less tax but have more public spending
>
> Health managers increasingly commission surveys that require employees or patients to agree or disagree with various statements about their perception of the organization. Can these questions be skilfully worded to give the answers the managers want to hear? How do staff or patients react when they can 'see through' the motives of the questionnaire and don't agree with its point of view?
>
> Consider a subject that most readers and politicians feel strongly about: taxation. Almost everyone believes they are being overtaxed and that taxation should be reduced; but at the same time everyone wants more money spent on health, education and crime prevention. One could argue that these ideas are not incompatible. For instance, the government could increase indirect taxation as opposed to income tax, to raise revenue while leaving people more discretion to spend as they wish.
>
> Or one could argue that 'the rich' should be heavily taxed, but not oneself. This 'politics-of-envy' thinking is very popular in Britain because whoever you are, you never include yourself among those to be taxed more highly.
>
> But alas the public are not so sophisticated. Various studies have shown that in opinion surveys people are contradictory. For example, an American polling company reported that 63% of people agreed with the view that: 'When 12,000 air-traffic controllers are willing to sacrifice their careers and economic security, and even go to jail, there must be some legitimate reasons for going on strike. The same poll found that 69% supported the opinion that: 'Since every air-traffic controller took an oath not to strike, President Reagan was right to fire them.' Obviously, a lot of people must have agreed with both statements, revealing nothing about whether they supported the strike. The writing of opinion items can therefore be highly political not good science unless done with best practice in mind.

The types of item to avoid are emotionally charged labels, including words such as 'thin' and 'fat', racist and sexist items and expressions, and any other potentially offensive statement. For example, *'After a Junior Doctor has completed* **his** *inspection of a patient, would you check as well?'* might be a reasonable survey question when investigating supervision, but it assumes that all Junior Doctors are male. The Researcher should use alternative expressions to avoid making assumptions that will alienate groups of Respondents.

Researchers should also avoid asking for the 'Christian name' instead of 'forename'.

Asking for highly personal information, such as income, poses a specially sensitive problem. It can usually be dealt with by providing a list of graded categories and asking the Respondent to choose the most appropriate.

Finally, it should be noted that questions must be written to avoid provoking both yes/no (agree/disagree) responses. *For example, 'Does the ambulance service need more ambulances and staff?'* Each question must be directed at a *singular* concept, either more ambulances or more staff.

Box 14 describes a less sophisticated but possibly quite powerful way of conducting surveys.

Box 14

Catchphrases versus standard survey questions?

One controversial solution to the writing of survey questions uses a familiar catchphrase to represent the issue. The formula 'X is a good/bad thing considering Y and Z' (agree or disagree?) is replaced by the simpler formula: 'X (good or bad?)'. This might tap immediate emotional reactions to controversial issues, and would be closer to actual behavioural dispositions.

The technique is to abandon the propositional form of an item, and instead simply present a list of brief labels or 'catchphrases' representing various familiar and controversial issues. It is assumed that, in the course of previous conversation and argument concerning these issues, the respondents have already placed themselves in relation to the general population, and are able to indicate their 'position' immediately and simply.

It is easy to demonstrate. Ask a group to write 5,000-word essays on capital punishment and have two judges assess whether they are, on balance, 'for' 'uncertain', or 'against'. Ask the essay-writer to complete the catchphrase poll as well. The results are nearly always identical and very little time and effort has been invested in the 'catchphrase' approach. Furthermore, this technique overcomes many of the problems of grammatical confusion and social desirability. Why not try it and see?

What follows is a simple economic beliefs scale:

Which of the following do you favour or believe in? Circle Yes or No. If absolutely uncertain, circle the question mark. There are no right or wrong answers. Do not discuss them; just give your first reaction.

Nationalization. YES   NO ?
Self-sufficiency. YES   NO ?
Socialism. YES   NO ?
Free market. YES   NO ?
Trade unions. YES   NO ?
Saving. YES   NO ?
Closed shops. YES   NO ?
Monetarism. YES   NO ?
Import controls. YES   NO ?
Privatization. YES   NO ?
Strikes. YES   NO ?
Informal black economy. YES   NO ?
Inheritance tax. YES   NO ?
Insurance schemes. YES   NO ?
Council housing. YES   NO ?
Private schools. YES   NO ?
Child benefits. YES   NO ?
Profit. YES   NO ?
Wealth tax. YES   NO ?
Public spending cuts. YES   NO ?

Scoring:
Odd items score Yes (3) ? (2) No (1)
Even items score Yes (1) ? (2) No (3)

Score 20 to 30 – you are probably very right wing.

(contd)

> Score 31 to 40 – you are probably a member of the entrepreneurial right.
> Score 41 to 50 – you are probably a supporter of New Labour.
> Score 51 to 70 – you are probably very left wing.
>
> Professional survey staff, management, pollsters, politicians and probably the Client would probably object to this method as its very simplicity and popularity seem to undermine its scientific basis. But Respondents would welcome its simplicity. This catch-phrase method may on occasion be superior to and simpler than more established methods.

Types of responses for survey items with forced choices

Responses to closed questions may take several forms, as listed below. What they have in common is that they all allow easy coding of the response so that they can be entered into a computer easily.

Yes/No responses

Yes and no responses are easy to score and analyse in terms of percentages. A third category (Don't know) can be added if the Respondent might have some difficulty in answering definitively. The disadvantages of this technique are that a misinterpretation of the question could lead to a response opposite to that intended, and asking for absolute responses may result in a refusal to answer. The binary data derived from such scales may also be more difficult to analyse using more complicated statistical procedures than simple percentages since dichotomous data generally require different and fairly advanced methodologies compared with scales having more than two response categories.

Checklist or nominal scale

A checklist or nominal scale provides Respondents with a series of alternative choices. They may tick (or circle) one or more options, depending on the choice available. A particular advantage of checklists is that they remind Respondents of some things that they might otherwise have forgotten. A good rule is to use either of the above methods when designing survey items that ask knowledge questions, such as the example given below:

Please tick where you are based:

USA 1
Europe 2
Elsewhere 3

Chapter 11 deals with the statistical analysis of nominal scales in some detail. However the important point is that this type of variable has severe limitations in terms of the type of statistics that can be applied to it.

The rating scale

With rating scales, the Respondent is required to make a quantitative judgement (i.e. give an opinion or make a subjective judgement), not just provide a yes/no response.

For example, the following statement could be rated:

'The ward kitchen is kept very clean' 1 2 3 4 5
(where the scale is as follows:

1. *Disagree strongly*
2. *Disagree*
3. *Neutral*
4. *Agree*
5. *Agree strongly).*

Category scales can also be used to summarize objective data because they still provide the Respondent with a limited choice of options. In relation to an objective scale of amount the Respondent is paid, the choice could be a series of boxes, each representing an income range on a linear scale:

less than £10,000   1
£10,001–£20,000   2
£20,001–£30,000   3
£30,001–£40,000   4

£40,001–£50,000   5
more than £50,000   6

Graphic scales are a type of rating scale particularly useful for measuring opinion. The response is marked not in a series of boxes but on a single line. The extremes of opinion are indicated at each end of the line, which is scaled uniformly into labelled divisions. Respondents are asked to mark their opinion with a cross. Typical scales are shown below:

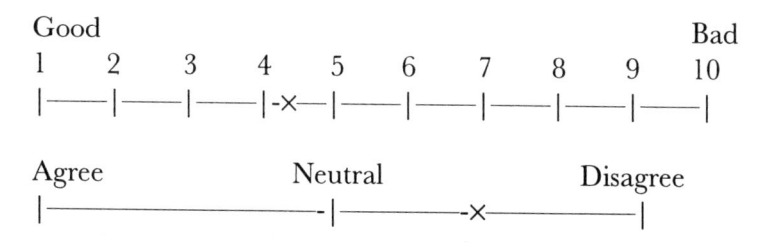

```
Good                                              Bad
 1    2    3    4    5    6    7    8    9    10
 |————|————|————|-x—|————|————|————|————|————|

Agree                  Neutral              Disagree
 |—————————————————-|—————————-x——————————|
```

Care should be taken to ensure that labels are placed as close as possible to the points they represent. If the same scale is used in different parts of the survey, the Researcher should ensure that the scale divisions remain the same. A problem that may arise is whether to score to the nearest marked point, or estimate the exact position. This matter tends to make the graphic scale difficult to score easily; therefore, in general, the standard rating scale is to be preferred.

Rank scales place a list of similar entities into order. For example:

(From the following list of five different uniform designs for physiotherapists, rank them in relation to your preference. The design you prefer most should be assigned the number 5, the design you prefer least should be assigned the number 1.

A list of the five different designs then follows).

A variation on this is to compare one named entity with others of the same genre, but not identified by name. For example:

Compare the furniture in the doctor's mess with that in other hospitals. Is it:

(1) Better than most
(2) About the same as most
(3) Not as good as most

Edwards, Thomas, Rosenfeld and Booth-Kewley (1997) provide a useful list of adjectives that can be used to describe points along a continuum. Here is an adapted selection of the most useful:

	1	2	3	4	5
Agreement	Strongly disagree	Disagree	Neither	Agree	Strongly agree
Frequency	Very dissatisfied	Dissatisfied	Neither	Satisfied	Very satisfied
Extent	No extent	Small extent	Moderate extent	Great extent	Very great extent

This type of scale is commonly found in surveys and questionnaires that measure attitudes and beliefs. The main advantages include (a) that it makes sense to the Respondent and therefore can easily be completed and (b) the ease with which fairly standard statistical methods can be applied (see Chapter 11).

Should there be a scale mid-point?

Whether or not a rating scale should have a scale mid-point is often the cause of controversy. Although there is not much difference in the quality of ratings obtained with or without a scale mid-point, evidence suggests that the use of a mid-point is more acceptable to Respondents because (a) it allows them to express a neutral attitude (b) it is less frustrating for Respondents as they are not forced into making a decision that they do not want to make, and (c) it allows proper interpretation of a scale mean that lies at the mid-point. Sometimes, however, it is a wise procedure to avoid a mid-point since the Client desires an answer in favour of or against a specific question and a 'Don't know' answer (i.e. a mid-point answer) is unacceptable.

Additive scales

Researchers are sometimes interested in the response to a single question that covers a whole content area. However, especially with regard to attitudes, there is usually the need to assess opinion on a group of items which collectively represent a content area.

For example, when attempting to measure the job satisfaction of members of the health professions, it would probably be better to measure the individual components of job satisfaction and then calculate the average. The kind of individual scales to be measured might include satisfaction with pay, promotion and lodgings, as well as many other facets of the job.

With this type of survey, it is necessary to combine the responses into a single entity. This is usually accomplished by taking the mean of the individual scores (see Chapter 11).

The procedure is:

(a) Set out the statements.
(b) Provide a rating of each statement, perhaps in terms of: Strongly agree, Agree, Neutral, Disagree, Strongly disagree (or some other appropriate group of phrases).
(c) Assign a numerical value to each response in terms of which statements are favourable and which are unfavourable (e.g. Very favourable = 2, Favourable = 1, Neutral = 0, Unfavourable = -1, Very unfavourable = -2).
(d) Compute the average score (as a general rule, never compare the total as there may be different numbers of items making up each of the content areas). See Chapter 11 for more information about calculating averages.

Formulating survey items in a clear and simple manner

It is absolutely essential that terms or expressions used in the questions are easily understood by the Respondents. When the concept underlying the question is simple, few difficulties are likely to arise. However, when the concept is more complex, for example relating to human attitudes and beliefs, greater care must be exercised in choosing an appropriate expression. Only terms that are widely used and have a generally accepted meaning should be employed. Colloquial expressions should, however, be avoided, because people who do not have English as a first language can find them difficult to understand.

For example, a poorly worded item in a survey could read:

'I felt like a fish out of water on my first day in the ward.'

This is a poor item because it is not specific about the reason why the Respondent may feel uncomfortable, and it also uses a colloquial expression that may not easily be understood by all people completing the survey. A better worded item could read:

'The other nurses often made me feel uncomfortable on my first day on the ward.'

And an even better version could read:

'The other nurses often made me feel anxious on my first day on the ward.'

Ensuring items are realistic

Difficulties may arise because Respondents are reluctant to answer questions; for example, they may feel embarrassed about a particular topic in the survey. *For example, a survey about people's history of sexually transmitted diseases will need careful and sensitive planning and implementation – otherwise there may be a danger of people faking answers or declining to take part in the survey.*

Alternatively Respondents may simply be unable to provide an answer, perhaps because it is outside their experience or because they have forgotten. Such circumstances may require changing the source of the data, or removal of the topic from the survey. *For example, it may be interesting to ask members of a health profession about whether they would prefer performance-related pay. However, without adequate preparation such questions may be outside the range of knowledge of the majority of Respondents.*

A good way of pre-empting these problems is to look at the distribution of answers obtained from your pilot study. If the percentage of respondents answering 'Don't know' or the amount of missing data is unduly large, then there is a problem with the current survey design.

Box 15 contains a list of items that measure lay people's beliefs about schizophrenia. You will see that the items are phrased so that the public's opinions about a very complex illness can be ascertained, even though their knowledge about the psychology and physiology of the illness may be minimal.

Box 15

Realistic questions for people to answer: Beliefs about Schizophrenia Questionnaire

Schizophrenia is an illness that even experts find difficult to understand. A questionnaire investigating lay people's beliefs about schizophrenia must translate many of the concepts and scientific jargon associated with such a complex illness into a clear and realistic questionnaire that can easily be understood by the public. Judge for yourself how well this was done.

Schizophrenia is caused by having blood relatives who are schizophrenic.

Schizophrenics have the right to be left alone as long as they do not break the law.

Mental hospitals are best used to remove schizophrenics from stressful homes to quieter settings.

Society has the right to protect people from schizophrenics.

Schizophrenics have the right to be treated as responsible adults.

The best way to treat schizophrenics is to respect their liberty and right to lead their own life.

There are more schizophrenics in some cultures and countries than others.

Schizophrenics have the right to personal freedom if they do not break the law.

The duty of society is to change and reduce the stresses and strains on schizophrenics and others.

Schizophrenic behaviour is so odd it shows how ill they are.

Whatever the aim of a mental hospital, it often ends up becoming a dumping ground for the poor and disadvantaged.

Schizophrenics have the right to be treated sympathetically.

Schizophrenia is caused by learning strange and bizarre behaviour from others.

Schizophrenics can be treated by punishing their bad behaviour.

Schizophrenic behaviour is symbolic of the problems encountered by the individual.

Making schizophrenics more responsible for their behaviour is the best way of treating them.

Mental hospitals are used to keep schizophrenics away from society.
Traumatic experiences in early childhood can cause schizophrenia.
Schizophrenics have the right to be released when their behaviour is acceptable to society.
Schizophrenics can be treated by making them act 'properly' by using rewards.
Stressful life events such as losing one's job can lead to schizophrenic behaviour.
Mental hospitals should act like correctional institutions (prisons).
The behaviour of schizophrenics is related meaningfully to their problems.
The best way to treat schizophrenics is with drugs.
The cause of schizophrenia is unusual early experience.
Mental hospitals sometimes end up simply providing shelter for the poor and other unfortunates.
Mental hospitals do little to get these people out of the hospital and back into society.
Schizophrenic behaviour is a way of dealing with the problems in the modern world.
Schizophrenia is caused by a chemical imbalance in the body.
It is society's duty to provide people and places to treat schizophrenics.
The behaviour of schizophrenics is an indication of a diseased mind.
The most effective way of helping schizophrenics is to create a society truly fit for them to live in.
The schizophrenic individual must cooperate fully with those treating him or her.
It is possible to help schizophrenics with long-term therapy with a trained counsellor.
Whatever the reason for the building of mental hospitals, they are often used to punish people who do not follow the rules of society.
A cause of schizophrenia is brain damage due to a virus.
Schizophrenic behaviour is nearly always bad and wrong.
The cause of schizophrenia is problems in emotional development as a child.
It is possible to help schizophrenics by simply talking to them about their problems.
A mental hospital is a kind of concentration camp, where people

(contd)

are subdued and degraded in order to make them easier to control.
It is possible to treat schizophrenics by surgery.
The schizophrenic has the duty to take responsibility for his or her actions and their outcomes.
It is the right of the schizophrenic to be cared for by society.
Producing a more comfortable and less stressful society is the best way to treat schizophrenics.
Schizophrenic behaviour is caused by harsh and unsympathetic treatment by others.
Privacy is the right of all schizophrenics.
Society has the duty to show sympathy to schizophrenics.
The best way to treat schizophrenics is to respect their right to lead their own lives.
Mental hospitals are often used to remove troublemakers from society.
The behaviour of schizophrenics is often sinful.
Society has the duty to respect the rights of the schizophrenic individual.
The behaviour of schizophrenics is a symptom of their illness.
Schizophrenics should not be judged morally for their actions, since they have little control over what they do.
Schizophrenia is caused by nothing more than problems in daily living.
The main function of the mental hospital is to provide an atmosphere for care and cure.
Schizophrenic behaviour is a result of dreadful treatment by other people.
Society has the duty to provide places where schizophrenics can go for help with their problems.
The most effective way of treating schizophrenics is to improve the society in which they live.
Mental hospitals should be used to teach schizophrenics to act responsibly so they can fit in with society.
Society has the right to punish or imprison those, like schizophrenics, whose behaviour breaks moral standards even if they do not break the law.
Treating people in an unpleasant manner can lead to schizophrenic behaviour.

> The way schizophrenics act is a 'code' which tells us about the way they are feeling.
> People are called schizophrenic when those around them can no longer cope with the way they behave.
> Schizophrenic behaviour often violates the moral rules by which we live.
> If lots of people treat someone badly, that person often displays schizophrenic behaviour.
> The function of the mental hospital is to rid society of those who threaten it.
> Most of the behaviour of schizophrenics is immoral.
> Schizophrenia is caused by learning from others with similar behaviour.
> A one-to-one relationship with a skilled therapist is the best way to treat schizophrenics.
> The cause of schizophrenia is the 'sick' society in which we live.
> Society has the duty to respect the liberty of the schizophrenic.
> The function of the mental hospital is to make the recovery of schizophrenics quicker.
> Schizophrenia is caused by a person's feeling guilty for his or her past actions.
> (From Furnham and Bower, 1992)

Eliminating bias

The Researcher must take great care to eliminate any possibility that the contents of the survey may affect the Respondents' views and expectations. If the Client insists on a biased survey to justify a position, then advise the Client that the exercise is pointless, meaningless and dangerous.

For example, a survey that is intended to provide support for a pay claim might include the following item:

'An increase in pay would make me more satisfied with my job'
whereas an item designed to provide support for a pay freeze might be:
'It would be wrong to ask for a pay award when the other members of the health professions have accepted a pay freeze'.

Equally, it is important to reduce the effect of Respondents' cheating or faking their answers to the survey or questionnaire. This is most commonly done by emphasizing the need to be honest during completion. See Box 16 for advice on how such 'liars' can be spotted.

Box 16

Spotting the liar in a questionnaire or survey

'The cheque is in the post.' 'Your CV will be kept on file.' Some things that people say are guaranteed to light up our internal lie detectors. But while some lies are easy to spot, others can be harder to identify from the replies given to surveys and questionnaires. There are four methods used to identify those Respondents who are determined to fake their answers in a questionnaire or survey:

1. Tell people not to lie. Let them know you expect lies, are used to them and hence are quite good at detecting them. This does not prevent exaggeration, subterfuge or selective memory loss, but it reduces many lies.
2. Have a lie scale. Answer these questions: 'Do you always wash your hands before a meal?'; 'Have you ever been late for an appointment?'; 'Have you ever taken the credit for something someone else did?' If someone answers Yes, No, No, he or she is a liar. Ask a few questions like these and see how people do. If they lie here, there is a fair chance they will lie on other questions as well.
3. Learn what to expect from a lie. Psychologists using this method administer the questionnaire to a group of Respondents who are asked to lie or who are known to be liars. This 'template' of answers can then be compared with a Respondent's replies to a survey to determine if there is any similarity between them.
4. Force them to make a choice. People will not usually admit to negative behaviour such as pilfering, politicking and backstabbing. One technique to elicit answers is to force them to say which they are most likely to do. You might ask: Are you likely to (i) make a private call on company time or (ii) take home company stationery? This forces candidates to admit the undesirable side of their nature.

> Liars can be relatively easily identified from the answers they provide to a survey. Catching liars is further simplified because Respondents believe that they can avoid being caught if they give consistent answers to similar questions. In fact, the only reason why questionnaires often ask many similar questions is to boost their reliability. But the more people believe that consistent answering is related to honest answering, the better it is for psychologists.
>
> Of course, in the end liars make their own punishment. Not only are they never believed, they also tend to judge others by their standards, so they can never believe anyone else!

Coding and data entry

Eventually all the information collected from each item will be entered into a spreadsheet in a computer for analysis (see Chapter 11). A good rule is to assign a count to each item on the survey answer-sheet that will be a new column in the spreadsheet so that it is easy to keep a track of the data entry.

For example, Question 11 in a survey could be concerned with determining the date of birth of the Respondent:

State date of birth:

Day	_____	*(34)*
Month	_____	*(35)*
Year	_____	*(36)*

Because the data are entered into separate columns of the spreadsheet (in this example columns 34, 35 and 36), the boxes are labelled on the survey to enable the person who enters the data to keep track of the data entry.

If the item was as follows:

I believe Junior Doctors work:
  (1) Too many hours per week
  (2) About right
  (3) Too few hours per week   *(35)*

then the score would only be entered in one column of the spreadsheet, and therefore just one spreadsheet column number (35) is specified by the survey designer.

Best practice in survey design means making the job easy and straightforward for Respondents. It is also good practice to enter the data into the spreadsheet in exactly the form expressed by the Respondents. If an item in the survey needs to be reverse-scored, then it should still be entered into the spreadsheet in a manner consistent with the Respondents' ratings and then recoded at a later stage.

Scanning hardware and software

It is possible to buy hardware and software that can scan, and then score, the survey automatically. Such equipment is relatively expensive but useful for data entry of results from large surveys (e.g. perhaps 1,000 or more Respondents answering more than 100 items each). There are definite pros and cons with the use of such hardware and software; expert advice should be sought before buying the equipment.

The internet offers not only easy questionnaire administration but also the capability of instant entry of data into a computer file by the Respondent who is answering the questions. For many Researchers, the cost and problems of designing an internet questionnaire or survey will be preferable to the greater problems of administration and scoring of pencil and paper administered versions.

Check, recheck and triple check

Finally, the Researchers should always check the survey for spelling and grammatical errors. They should have the items reviewed by several colleagues because surveys can never be checked enough prior to printing. The more time the Researcher spends designing the survey, the greater the chance of small errors creeping in – simply because the Researcher is so familiar with the material that he or she might miss details.

Writing the survey

Summary

The Researcher should:

(a) Plan the size and structure of the survey or questionnaire
(b) Be very clear, precise and unbiased when writing survey items.
(c) Recognize the difficulties involved in analysis when asking open questions.
(d) Choose between 'Yes'/'No' answers, checklist answers and rating scales when using closed items.
(e) Understand how to average the items from one content area to calculate a summary score.
(f) Make the data entry task easy by coding the survey.
(g) Think about using hardware and software to make data entry automatic.
(h) Put the time and effort into checking that the survey will work.

Part 4:
Evaluating the items

Chapter 10
The pilot study

Introduction

Related items in a survey should be clear and understandable. However they must also be consistent (reliable), meaningful (valid), and provide a spread of scores so that they are able to discriminate between Respondents. By following the guidelines set out in this book, the Researcher has already found out how to design items that should meet these criteria. This chapter provides guidelines on ways of statistically checking whether these criteria have been met before carrying out the actual survey itself.

The following guidelines are recommended:

(a) For simple surveys which aim to collect factual data, conduct a **qualitative analysis** as outlined below;
(b) For complex surveys, especially those which seek opinions from Respondents, conduct a **qualitative and quantitative analysis** as outlined below. Inexperienced Researchers are strongly advised to seek expert advice as the statistics used to analyse the items using quantitative methods will be confusing.

Qualitative approaches to the trial run

For simple surveys that do not seek opinions but facts, this qualitative approach is sufficient on its own. Researchers should follow one of the processes listed below:

(a) 'Think aloud' survey development. On a one-to-one basis, survey designers sit down with a range of people from target groups and ask them to 'think aloud' (to express verbally what they are thinking) as they respond to each of the items. This detects if people are misinterpreting a particular item, and why they are misinterpreting it. It may be that different groups perceive, interpret and respond to the items in different ways.

(b) Small-group discussion in which group members discuss the survey as a whole, as well as individual items. The group usually consists of people who have taken the test, or a group of experts in a particular area. Membership of the group is determined by the needs and interests of the survey developer. However, the group should be critical, informed and representative of the group to be surveyed.

Quantitative analysis methods to trial attitude surveys

When the Researcher wishes to investigate attitudes, then a pilot analysis or trial run is also necessary. Once the draft of the survey has been administered to a representative group of Respondents, it remains for the survey developer to analyse scores and responses to individual items. The different types of statistical scrutiny that the survey data can potentially undergo at this point are referred to collectively as item analysis. Researchers *must* understand how the data are to be analysed prior to conducting a trial study.

The trial study

Having created a pool of items from which the final version of the survey will be developed, the Researcher should administer it to people similar to those for whom the survey was designed. Thus, for example, if a survey is designed to measure the effect of a specific exercise for pregnant mothers, it would be inappropriate to test the survey on men! Equally important is the number of people to be included in the trial study. The appropriate number depends upon the size of the final survey; for many purposes 50 people will be optimal, although less may be sufficient. The main point is that the Researcher should keep survey conditions of the trial study as close as possible to those under which the actual survey will be conducted. It is also a good idea for the Researcher to ask Respondents to report their reactions to, and criticisms of, the survey after they have completed it.

Item analysis of opinion-based surveys

A trial is evaluated by looking at the items in the survey in terms of item quality and overall validity and reliability. Reliability provides a measure of the consistency of the information obtained, and validity measures the accuracy of the information itself. (See Anastasi, 1988; Kline, 1993; Kline, 1986 and Rust and Golombok, 1989 for further information about the psychometrics of surveys and questionnaires.)

Among the tools that Researchers might employ to analyse and select items are indexes of:

(a) an item's facility and difficulty (or response distribution)
(b) an item's discriminability
(c) reliability
(d) validity.

Item facility

Item facility is an index of the number of responses in each category out of the total number of responses made to a particular item. For example, 25% of Respondents might answer 'Yes' and 75% might answer 'No' to a particular item in a survey.

In an objective survey, items in which a large proportion of people tick the same box are useful because they provide essential information (e.g. 78% of staff are male). However, there is little point in recording attitudinal results that do not show differences between Respondents, since the whole purpose of the scale is usually to show these differences. *For example, there is little point in including an item in which most people rate themselves as extrovert, since extroversion is merely the opposite pole of introversion as defined by the differences between people.*

An index of the facility of the 'average' item for a particular survey can be calculated by averaging the item-facility indices for all the survey's items (total number of items on the survey). For items with two response categories, a good average is approximately 50%, with individual items on the survey ranging in difficulty from about 20% to 80% in one of the categories.

Further analysis to be undertaken would involve plotting the distribution. Look for possible ceiling or floor effects. Is the distribution single peaked or double (or more) peaked. Such effects may be pointers to subtle problems with items, which can be solved by rewording. *For example, 'Do you always wash before a meal?' would be an* item which is likely to be severely skewed towards one end of the scale; 'Do you sometimes wash before a meal?' is likely to be much less skewed.

Item discriminability

Measures of item discrimination indicate how adequately an item separates or discriminates between high scorers and low scorers in general. Common sense dictates that an item is not doing its job if it is answered positively by Respondents who in general have a negative attitude.

The appropriate index is the correlation of the item score versus the total of the attitude score to determine how much of a contribution it makes to the overall score (see Chapter 11 for the information about correlations).

For example, if the following items had a positive correlation with the total of a scale of management ability:

(a) Knows how to handle subordinates
(b) Always knows what to do
(c) Has charisma
(d) Has authority

but the following had virtually a zero correlation:

(e) Leads from the front
(f) Is well dressed

then the survey designer should reject items (e) and (f) because they are inadequate components of the scale.

The overall evaluation of the survey

Reliability

Once the good items have been selected at the expense of the poor items, the Researcher can assess reliability of the survey by measuring the item reliability index. The item reliability index provides an indication of the internal consistency of an attitude scale; the higher this index, the greater the test's internal consistency. Cronbach's Alpha is a widely reported measure of internal consistency (see Chapter 11). A good rule of thumb is that each attitude scale should have a value of about 0.7 or more.

For example, the content areas of a scale of management may have consisted of the following items:

(a) Knows how to handle subordinates
(b) Always knows what to do
(c) Has charisma
(d) Has authority
(e) Leads from the front
(f) Is well dressed

It may be that Cronbach's Alpha is low if the scale includes items (e) and (f), but much higher if the scale does not contain items (e) and (f). In this case, such a result would be a reconfirmation of the item discriminability analysis.

Validity of the scale

Validity is all about whether the questionnaire or survey performs in the way that it should do or is claimed to do. It is easy, therefore, to see that this is perhaps the most fundamental component of preparing a survey or questionnaire for use. *For example, a test of nursing knowledge should measure knowledge obtained during training as opposed to measuring academic qualifications, age, job satisfaction, motivation, etc.*

However, all this is easier said than done. The concept of nursing knowledge, for example, is somewhat difficult to define and without a clear definition of the criterion (i.e. the dependent measure or that which we are desiring to measure when constructing the scale), it is difficult to determine the validity. In fact, a questionnaire or survey is usually used precisely because the subject area is difficult to define. Most Researchers would agree that if they could define and measure the criterion properly then they would do that and not use a survey or questionnaire at all!

Our discussion of validity breaks down into the following areas:

Face validity

The issue of face validity is both crucial and irrelevant at the same time (see Box 17). Face validity concerns whether the survey or questionnaire *appears* to be measuring what it says it does. To the lay person (such as the Respondents and perhaps even the Client) this is a crucial issue. Respondents are unlikely to be happy to complete a survey that seems to make no sense and the Client will mistrust the results of such a survey. This is true even when the questions are valid.

For example, a Researcher developed a test of anxiety for use in staff selection. Theoretically valid questions may include 'Are you afraid of creepy crawly insects?' 'Are you scared of snakes?' 'Do you look at your tongue in the morning?' Such questions are theoretically valid because theories of anxiety suggest high scorers have phobias about insects and reptiles and may well be hypochondriacs. Nevertheless, if these items are presented to a candidate for a job as an administrator within a dental surgery there seems to be no direct link between these questions and the job for which the person is applying. However, it also seems reasonable to ask questions about anxiety since people low on anxiety may be supposed to be higher performers than those high on anxiety.

Thus it may be supposed that questions of high face validity are crucial. After all, it is still possible to ask questions about anxiety while maintaining high face validity. Questions like this could include: 'Would you get anxious dealing with members of the public?' 'Do you generally feel well enough to come to work?' The problem with these questions is that the correct answer is easy to guess. Any candidate should be able to work out how to answer questions of high face validity in order to be a high scorer.

We conclude that high face validity is a definite problem with questionnaires or surveys when Respondents have something to gain by faking their answers (either positively or negatively). However, for anonymous surveys or other types of surveys where Respondents may have little to gain through faking, high face validity is useful because the Respondents and the Client will have greater faith in the instrument.

Box 17

Face validity: Why people's judgements of validity are inaccurate

Furnham (1994) asked why people have a habit of believing in, consulting and acting upon the advice of bogus alternative practitioners. It seems that the answer may be similar to why people believe in graphology and astrology, practices whose predictions contrast with the scientific method and have a highly dubious record in terms of validity.

> For a long time, psychologists have been investigating the possibility that horoscopes and handwriting analyses have some validity, but none of significance has ever been reported. Yet people from all backgrounds still believe in astrology and graphology. The same is true of the more outlandish cults in alternative and complementary medicine. It seems likely that research into astrology can tell us something about why patients believe in bogus medicine.
>
> Paradoxically, the most likely reason for the popularity of graphology and astrology is that they are true. However, the reason why they are true is that they are vague, positive generalizations that are generally true of most people and yet are derived specifically for a named individual. Psychologists refer to this as the Barnum effect; named after Phineas T. Barnum, a showman and circus owner in nineteenth-century America who claimed 'There's a sucker born every minute' and whose formula for success was 'A little something for everybody'. It seems that people believe in astrology and graphology because they take generalized, positive descriptions, which are true of most people, to be specifically true of themselves.
>
> Research suggests that the Barnum effect provides an explanation for the popularity of the more exotic forms of complementary and alternative medicine. It seems that people believe in bogus branches of alternative medicine because they are given bland, psychological and biological feedback that is, in fact, true of everybody. It can be concluded from this kind of work that the validity of a study cannot be investigated by a study of the beliefs of the subjects since their opinion can easily be swayed to the positive by careful feedback. It is best to seek evidence of validity elsewhere as opposed to relying on face validity.

Predictive validity

A survey or questionnaire has predictive validity if it has the capacity to predict some other object (usually referred to as a criterion). Predictive ability is usually regarded as one of the most important features of a questionnaire or survey because it suggests that it can measure some external and unconnected phenomenon.

The problem with the predictive validity stems from the problem of identifying a good criterion against which the efficacy of the survey or questionnaire can be measured. At first thought, this seems easy. A selection questionnaire could be compared with yearly performance; a survey investigating the comfort of a new type of office seat could be compared with office worker's comfort ratings; a patient health survey could be compared with expert clinician evaluations. All this seems straightforward, and yet it rarely is.

The problems stem from inappropriateness and the difficulty in measuring meaningful criteria. Often, criteria are not as appropriate as is first thought. Yearly performance can be a poor criterion as a result of inappropriateness because there is annual variation in staff performance due to a variety of relatively irrelevant reasons (e.g. pregnancy, moving house, amount of team support, gaining or losing clients, changing boss) and because it is difficult to measure staff performance anyhow. Sales figures or percentage of target met can be too simplistic to really reflect sales performance – and sales seems to be a job that is very easy to measure using objective criterion measures. Annual appraisals are often used but these are often flawed as a result of difficulty of measurement such as rater errors (e.g. leniency, halo and central tendency) as explained further in Box 18.

We conclude that predictive validity is an extremely important measure of validity but that Researchers need to understand the problems of its measurement that usually occur as a result of poor criteria.

Box 18

Common types of rating error

There are many problems associated with ratings, and the kind of rating errors that Respondents make when completing a survey or questionnaire include the following:

1. Halo Effect
This can be either positive or negative. What it means is that people assume that good and bad characteristics in the questionnaire go together. Thus they are unable to rate the content areas identified by the Researcher as being as independent of each other as was supposed.

Let us consider a few examples outside the world of surveys to see how this works in practice. For example:

- Men have been known to hire secretaries more for their looks than their typing ability. They assume that attractiveness means they will be efficient at word processing; clearly this is not always the case.
- Attractive men and women are more likely to get lower prison sentences. Being attractive means being good.
- The time mental patients stay in hospital is often directly related to how attractive/ugly they are. Here the hospital administrator commits the halo error by confusing physical attractiveness with 'sanity'.
- People wear ties, scarves and other badges to show which school they went to, hoping that this will influence people they meet. If you went to a good school some people naturally assume that you are good at everything. This is another example of the halo effect.

The danger of the halo effect is that people are thought of as generally good, average and bad, rather than recognized as being good at some things and not others.

2. Fixing the system
Some people attempt to manipulate or cheat the survey or questionnaire by giving all positive scores. For example, this might be done on an appraisal form to ensure their subordinates get high scores (perhaps to get them more pay). This usually does not work because departmental differences can be checked, compared and normalized. Moreover, when Respondents attempt to fix the system, they are not providing the decision makers with the right information and can dangerously undermine the whole system. To continue with the example, managers need to tell their staff what they are doing wrong and right, not bribe them. They will be caught and the employees may feel more unhappy than if they had been told the truth in the first place.

3. Fear of negative reactions
Some people believe that accurate completion of a questionnaire or survey may be demotivating because it may involve too much criticism without advice on how things could be done better. Others

(contd)

may be extremely harsh when completing a questionnaire or survey even though this does not reflect their true feelings, simply because they are unhappy (perhaps in their treatment by the organization).

4. Personal bias theories
Some people have personal, sometimes rather odd theories about human nature. Muhammad Ali once said in a talk that people are like *fruit*. Some fruit are hard on the outside and some are soft. This leaves the following pattern: the *walnut* is 'hard on the outside, but soft on the inside'; the *prune*, 'soft on the outside and hard on the inside'; the *pomegranate*, 'hard on the inside and the outside', and the *grape*, 'soft on the inside and the outside'. Respondents have their own sometimes rather eccentric theories that they apply to surveys and questionnaires. No wonder there can sometimes be problems of reliability!

5. Memory deficits
People forget their own behaviour and that their memory is often distorted. If you do something well nobody remembers; if you do something badly nobody forgets. Respondents may need to keep *notes* about good and bad behaviours so that they can remember specific facts

6. Projection
Some people see things in other people that they are afraid to see in themselves. They project their anxiety and anger on to others, seeing them as lazy, incompetent, full of gossip, unmotivated, etc., whereas they are the ones who have these characteristics. Thus surveys and questionnaires may not be measuring real opinions, attitudes and beliefs.

7. Attribution errors
People may see themselves as being very variable and inconsistent, but raters may well see just consistency. Ask people if they are an introvert or extrovert and they say neither or both. Ask them about their boss, spouse, etc., and they will say that he or she is definitely an introvert or extrovert. This means that people strive too hard to look for consistency in others while not finding it in themselves. They look for consistently good or bad characteristics, whereas the reality is that people have both at the same time.

Concurrent validity

A survey or questionnaire will have concurrent validity if it correlates with another test (the criterion test) that measures the same subject area. This is a straightforward way of assessing the validity of a new instrument except for the following non-trivial problems:

- Why develop a new instrument if an old instrument is so good that it can be used as a criterion? Basically, the new questionnaire or survey must have special qualities (such as that it is shorter or less easy to fake) than the criterion questionnaire for there to be sufficient reason to develop a new questionnaire.
- If there is no satisfactory criterion instrument against which to compare the new questionnaire or survey, then what is the point of correlating them together since the correlation is not easy to understand? A low correlation could be interpreted as showing that the criterion test is flawed; equally a high correlation could show that both tests are flawed in the same ways. All that can be said is that evidence of concurrent validity adds to our knowledge of validity but on its own is of limited use.

Content validity

A questionnaire or survey is said to have content validity if it covers the domain of content areas of the subject in question. Thus a survey investigating the culture of a hospital would need to cover the full range of constructs that go together to measure culture. Usually, content validity is demonstrated by expert evaluation and critique of the instrument. It should be noted that this is a different form of validity to face validity since the evaluation is performed by experts who evaluate the questionnaire or survey in terms of its content as opposed to what the content appears to be like.

Construct validity

This final form of validity sets out to determine if it is possible, through knowledge of the questionnaire or survey content, to derive hypotheses that when supported would show evidence of validity. It is important to note that hypotheses can also be derived that set out to determine what is *not* measured as well as what is measured.

For example, a Researcher wishes to determine the construct validity of a learning difficulties test. The following hypotheses are formulated that, if proven, would provide reasonably strong evidence in favour of the questionnaire:

- *Scores will correlate with other measures of learning difficulty*
- *Scores will negatively correlate with academic performance*
- *Scores will negatively correlate with teacher evaluation*
- *High scorers and low scorers will be differentially found in different occupational groups.*

Moreover the Researcher also formulates some hypotheses that, if disproven, would support the validity of the questionnaire:

- *The questionnaire will not be related to any of the major traits of personality*
- *The questionnaire will not be related to social class.*

Of course, the reader will be able to think of many more hypotheses that will seek to prove the construct validity of a questionnaire such as that described above. It is never possible to provide complete evidence in favour of a questionnaire or survey, but it is possible to demonstrate reasonable evidence.

To summarize, the Researcher should assess validity in the following manner:

(a) **Face validity:** Desirable unless Respondents may be likely to fake their answers.
(b) **Predictive validity:** This can be assessed by measuring the predictive accuracy of the survey. For example, if the objective of the survey was to measure job satisfaction, then an examination of subsequent results should predict turnover, absenteeism, number of grievances, etc.
(c) **Concurrent validity:** This requires a comparison between scores with the new survey and a well established one; alternatively, a comparison can be made with the judgement of an expert committee. In both situations a high correlation indicates concurrent validity.
(d) **Content validity:** This refers to the accuracy with which the questions adequately represent the qualities they are presumed to measure. It is usually established by referring to an expert committee.

(e) Construct validity: This is found when hypotheses derived from theory are supported by the results of survey or questionnaire.

For example, a Researcher is designing a survey that measures attitude to smoking within the health professions. High scorers are anti-smoking whereas low scorers are pro-smoking. The survey could be validated by measuring:

(1) Predictive validity by determining how well it predicts current number of cigarettes smoked.
(2) Concurrent validity by determining whether results of this survey correlate with the results of other smoking questionnaires.
(3) Content validity by determining if a panel of experts agree that the items can measure attitude towards smoking.
(4) Construct validity by determining if various hypotheses about attitude to smoking are supported. For example, it is possible that high scorers will have more positive attitudes towards restriction of smoking in public places.

Predictive validity and concurrent validity are often measured by means of correlations, which are described in Chapter 11.

Relationship between validity and reliability

A questionnaire or survey that has little consistency (i.e. that has little reliability) is unlikely to posses high validity because something that does not produce the same score twice is unlikely to be related to anything else. However the converse is not necessarily true. A questionnaire or survey with high reliability (i.e. it will consistently produce the same score) may not be valid simply because it is measuring the incorrect variable or is measuring the appropriate variable but in an inappropriate manner.

Summary

The Researcher should:

(a) Conduct a qualitative trial run if designing a 'fact' based survey.
(b) Conduct a qualitative and quantitative trial run if designing an 'opinion' based survey.

(c) Use a quantitative survey to ensure that the items differentiate between Respondents, discriminate between high and low scorers in general and have internal consistency.
(d) Use a quantitative survey to ensure that the survey has adequate validity and reliability.

Part 5: Analysing the results

Chapter 11
Analysing data from surveys

Introduction

An analysis of the results of a survey or questionnaire is performed to make the results understandable to the Client and other interested parties. Without using statistics, the Researcher would not be able to reduce and summarize the data so that meaningful conclusions can be drawn and communicated.

This is not a statistics text and in an era when most analyses are performed by computer it is unnecessary to dwell too long on the maths needed to understand statistical principles and how to actually calculate statistics by hand. Instead the emphasis of this chapter is to introduce the basic statistics used to analyse data so that the Researcher and those who read the final report will have a clear sense of direction. We believe that all Researchers should have the necessary skills to be able to perform a basic analysis of the data, whether they are good at maths or not. To be able to analyse data requires logical thinking, the ability to learn and develop one's repertoire of techniques, basic arithmetic skills, a good computer and a good statistics software package.

Analysis of surveys will be straightforward if four simple rules are followed:

1. Plan the analysis. The Researcher *must* plan what is to be done while designing the survey or questionnaire and must never commit to a specific survey design without prior thought about the analysis of the data.
2. Researchers must *never* do analyses which are beyond their experience.

3. Researchers must *never* rely on computer packages to make sense of what they do not understand. Knowledge and experience is crucial when it comes to using computer packages to avoid the 'garbage in, garbage out' problem.
4. Researchers must *never* expect experts to be able to do this part without having been involved in the planning of the survey. Once Researchers have got this far on their own, then the chances are that they will have to finish the survey on their own. If Researchers are then unable to perform the appropriate statistical analyses, or worse still, get them wrong, then the whole project will fail.

When the survey has been completed and all the questionnaires have been returned, attention must be directed to analysing the results. The first step is to understand the nature of the data that is to be analysed (see Box 19). Then, as the second step, data need to be broken down into tallies (frequency of a particular response), averages, relationships, comparisons, and/or trends.

Box 19

Types of measurement found in surveys and questionnaires

Nominal

Nominal scales are scales where the number attached to each category has no meaning in its own right and is used purely for descriptive purposes. *For example, gender of respondent might be coded as 0 for Male and 1 for Female. This coding does not imply that Females are larger or better by 1 unit than Males but simply implies that there is a difference in the two categories. It may also be that different surgeries or different hospitals are coded as 1, 2, 3, or 4. Again this is purely for descriptive use and does not necessarily imply that there are quantitative differences between them on a scale of 1 to 4.*

Ordinal/Rank

An ordinal or rank scale exists if the numbers attached to a scale indicate how the categories can be ordered on a particular variable. *For example, it may be that patients are classified into those which are private (1) and those which are public (0). In this case there is a dimension – perhaps quality of service — which is reflected by this classification. Private patients may receive better quality of service than public patients and thus can be ranked higher than private patients. However, it is not possible to say precisely how much better that service is.*

Another example. Doctors may classify night calls according to their priority as follows: (2) Attend straight away (1) Advise the patient comes to the clinic (0) Provide advice on the telephone. The dimension being rated is severity of symptoms reported where 2 is the most serious, 1 is moderately serious and 0 is the least serious. However, it is not possible to see precisely how much difference there is between the different categories, except to say that they can be ranked.

Interval

An interval scale exists if the categories on a dimension not only can be ranked but the size of the difference between categories can be quantified. *For example, the size of a hospital could be categorized on a three-point scale (large, medium, small) for auditing purposes according to number of staff, numbers of patients, surface area, etc. Here the scale categories are defined to have a known interval between them.*

Strictly speaking, most psychological scales are interval in nature since we cannot say precisely what the interval between the scale categories is. However, most experts are prepared to make a few assumptions in order to treat rating scales and other psychological scales as interval scales. Thus a Researcher may develop a questionnaire designed to investigate coping styles. Respondents can score between 1 and 10, where 10 implies optimal coping strategies. Here we know that the bigger the number, the better the coping, so it is at least an ordinal scale. However, most experts would tend to regard the scale as having near-to-interval properties and so it can be treated as such. Clearly, the better the scale design and the more attention paid to developing equidistant intervals between category definitions, the more the scale is likely to have interval characteristics.

Ratio

This type of scale is an interval scale which can be objectively anchored. Thus the a non-category scale of number of employees is a ratio scale because 0 employees is an objective anchor to the scale. Many scales that have a physical identity are ratio scales, whereas few psychological scales are ratio scales.

Selecting analysis methods

The appropriate analysis method is dependent on the objectives, who is surveyed, the design of the survey, the type of data collected, and the audience for the survey results. There are five important questions that must be considered:

(a) How many people were surveyed?
Certain analysis methods (e.g. t-tests and ANOVA) require larger samples than others (e.g. Mann-Whitney). However, tallies, averages, and measures of variation can often be used on even quite small numbers (but never less than about 30).

(b) Is the survey looking for relationships or associations? To describe a single variable, then tallies, averages and measures of variation are suitable. The relationship between two variables (e.g. attitude to authority and age) can be analysed using the Pearson product-moment correlation provided continuous data are available. However, when the data are in the form of ranks, the Spearman rank-order statistic is used.

(c) Will the survey be comparing groups? When comparing groups, the Mann-Whitney U, t-test, ANOVA, chi-square, and others are useful in determining whether differences are due to a real occurrence, or result from chance, or some other effect. Although they are easily calculated, many undergraduates struggle for years to understand these tests and how to interpret their results. Just because a Researcher can work out how to compute these statistics does not mean that they have been compiled correctly or interpreted correctly.

(d) Will the survey be conducted once or several times? This will depend on whether the survey design is cross-sectional or longitudinal (i.e. seeking descriptions or trends). The dependent t-test and repeated measures ANOVA may help to determine whether the results are meaningful.

(e) Are the data recorded as numbers and percentages, or scores and averages? Data recorded as numbers and percentages (categorical data) may be analysed using chi-square; when recorded as scores or averages (continuous data) ANOVA is likely to be more appropriate.

Descriptive statistics

The most commonly used analytical tools are:

(a) Numbers (e.g. tallies, frequencies, percentages, and cross-tabulations). Many survey reports just present the percentage of response to certain key questions. This in fact has many advantages over more complex methods. The method is simple for the Researcher, simple for the Client to understand, meaningful in the sense that the results represent the data, and powerful in the sense that the results can be presented graphically in a forceful manner that makes a clear point. Plainly, the disadvantage of presenting results purely in terms of percentages is that so much more is missed than if the results were analysed with greater sophistication.
(b) Averaging (e.g. the mean, median, and mode)
(c) Measures of variation (e.g. range and standard deviation).

The following example illustrates these statistical methods. One question in a survey sent out to 50 nurses working in a liver transplant ward asked how likely they thought it was that they might catch an infection whilst at work over the next two years. Responses were on a 10-category rating scale where a high score indicated a high likelihood of catching an infection. The following responses were obtained:

5	4	5	7	3	4	4	7	5	9
5	3	5	7	4	5	6	8	5	2
6	5	6	7	5	8	5	5	1	7
7	7	7	8	4	8	5	4	2	6
5	9	8	2	5	9	8	3	4	6

Very little can be made of this set of results just by visually inspecting them in their raw form. It is important therefore to summarize the main features of the results so that they can be better understood.

Tallies or frequency counts

This analysis works well when the Respondents are presented with a list and asked to tick the item closest to their own views. The tally or frequency count is a computation of how many Respondents make a particular choice and the results can then be given as a number or as a percentage.

Before using the example above, let us take a more simple case in which there is just a choice of two answers.

For example, if there is an item in a questionnaire:
'I am likely to leave in 5 years' 'Yes' 'No'

then results could be reported as: *55% said they were unlikely to leave in 5 years whereas 45% reported that they were.* Plainly, the simple percentage of response to a certain category can be a very straightforward means of summarizing the results of a survey.

Now let's go back to our 'liver ward' example. The first thing to do is to create a frequency distribution which is a systematic arrangement of responses from the smallest to the largest, together with a tally of the number of times that response was made. We arrange the 50 ratings made by the fictitious nurses in order, and note the frequency with which each rating has been made.

The frequency distribution is easily calculated by hand by simply determining how many scores are associated with each score – this is the frequency or tally and is shown in Table 3. Note how they are ordered from smallest to largest; that each category does not overlap with any of the others; and that all the scores can be accommodated in the categories that have been chosen. The total of the frequencies is 50.

Table 3. Frequency of ratings of chance of infection from working in a liver transplant ward

Score	Frequency	Percent	Cumulative per cent
1	1	2	2
2	3	6	8
3	3	6	14
4	7	14	28
5	14	28	56
6	5	10	66
7	8	16	82
8	6	12	94
9	3	6	100
Total	50	100	100

Now it is easy to see the lowest score and the highest score, and it is becoming easier to understand the characteristics of the distribution of the variable (such as where most of the scores lie and what was the most common score). Prior to the construction of Table 3 it would not have been possible to understand the data in this way.

Often the percentage of the total is also calculated as shown in Table 3. Percentages are calculated by means of the simple formula:

% of response = (frequency of response in a category/total sample size) * 100

Thus the percentage of nurses who made a rating of 4 is 7/50 * 100 = 14%.

The percentage of nurses that made a rating in each category of the rating scales is shown in Table 3. The total of the per cents must equal 100, so this is a useful check when the calculations are performed by hand. The frequencies or the percentages can be plotted as a histogram to create a chart of high visual impact (see Figure 3). Now it is very easy to understand the data.

The shape of the distribution is usually of great interest to the Researcher. Symmetrical distributions are found if, when folded

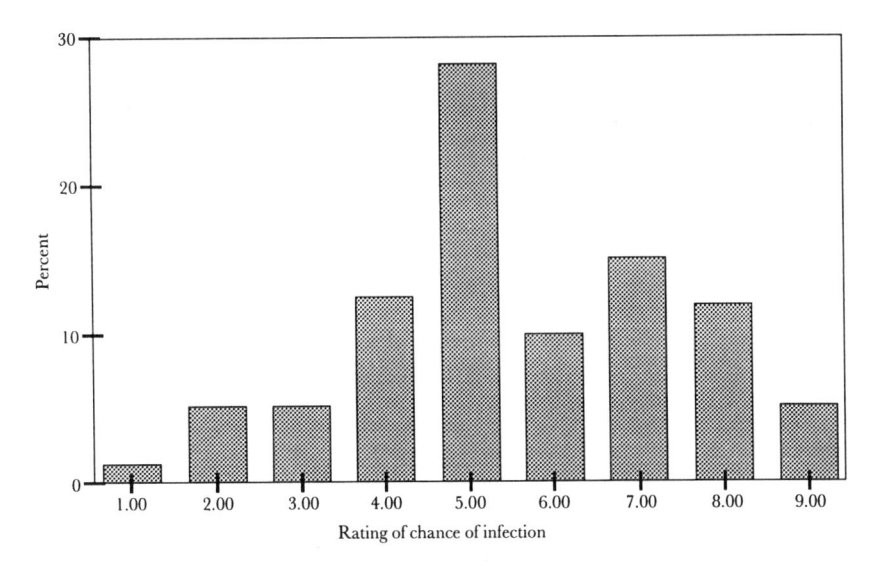

Figure 3. Histogram of nurses' rating of the chances of infection from working in a liver transplant ward.

over, the two halves can be superimposed on each other with only minor discrepancies. The most commonly found symmetrical distribution has a bell-shaped curve (known as the normal distribution). Here the highest frequency of occurrence is found in the middle of the scale, and the frequencies diminish symmetrically towards each end of the scale in the shape of a bell. Many physiological scales (e.g. size, weight or length of a pregnancy) and psychological (e.g. intelligence, extroversion) scales follow approximate bell-shaped curves. The data shown in Figure 3 are not too far off a bell-shaped distribution although there are discrepancies (especially in the '6' category of the rating scale, where a far larger percentage could have been expected if a normal distribution was being followed).

Asymmetrical distributions are skewed because the highest score is not at the centre of the scale. Consequently one end of the distribution has a longer tail than the other. A good example would be income of health professionals. The majority of staff have low to moderate incomes with a few people on high incomes. The shape of the distribution would reflect this, with the highest frequencies of income being relatively low with a tail (i.e. low frequencies) towards high incomes.

Respondents will also often comment on the modality of the distribution. Unimodal distributions have just one peak whereas multimodal distributions have two or more peaks. *For example, the canteen manager of a hospital can predict that the frequency of use of the canteen will follow a trimodal distribution during the working day as staff arrive for breakfast, lunch and dinner. During other times of the day, the use of the canteen is likely to be far less. Multimodal distributions are relatively rare but must be identified when they occur.*

A further step is also often useful. This is to calculate the cumulative frequency distribution as also shown in Table 3. This is simply the sum of the percentages that have achieved a certain category. Thus 2% of nurses provide a rating of 1 and 6 % of nurses provide a rating of 2. Therefore 2+6 = 8% of nurses provide a rating of 2 or less. Or 2+6+6+14+28+10 = 66% of nurses provide a rating of 6 or less. The cumulative frequency distribution is a powerful way of providing further insight into the data, especially when it is important to determine the percentage of people who achieve a certain score or less. For example, it may be considered that above a rating of 6 the morale of the nurses will be severely damaged. Using the cumulative frequency distribution we can say that 66% of nurses have a score equal to, or less than, 6 and 44% (i.e. 100 - 66) have a score of more than 6. The cumulative frequency distribution of the nurses is shown graphically in Figure 4.

Averages: means, medians and modes

Frequency distributions are useful for determining a pattern of responses amongst a group. Often, however, even this is too detailed a picture and a simpler summary is more useful. Usually, Researchers want to produce a simple number that represents a group. The appropriate measure of central tendency (mean, median or mode) is the best single summary of a group because it represents the most typical category of response. For use with a nominal scale the appropriate measure is the mode; the median may be used for ranked scales and the mean is generally used with interval, ratio and rating scales. An exception to this rule is when the distribution of an interval, ratio or rating scale is skewed. Here the median is likely to be the most useful measure of central tendency.

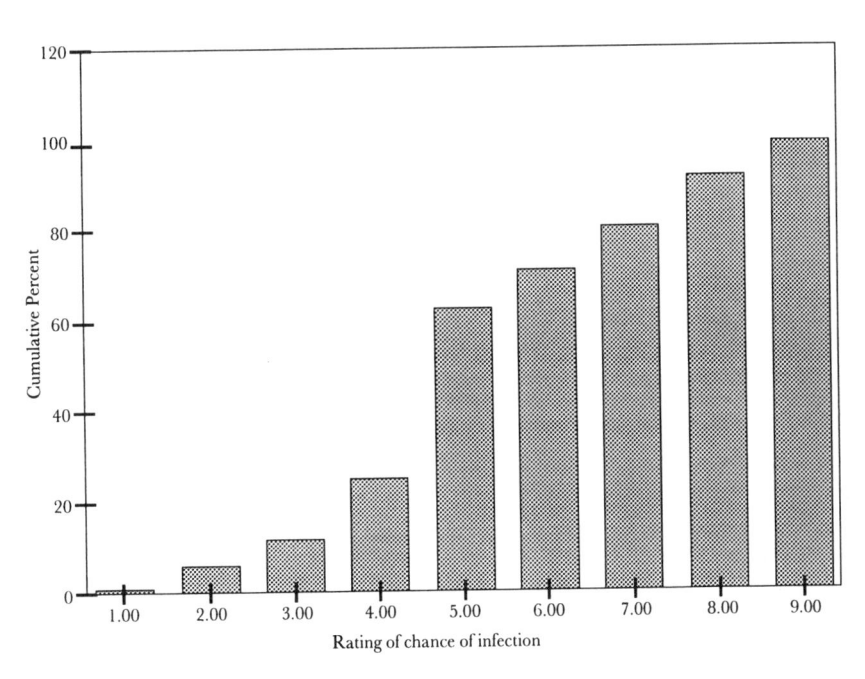

Figure 4. Cumulative frequency distribution of nurses' ratings of the chance of infection when working in a liver transplant ward.

The mean

The mean is the most commonly used measured of central tendency and is calculated from the following equation:

$$\text{Mean} = \frac{\Sigma x}{N}$$

where Σx = the sum of all the individual values and N is the number of values.

For example, it might be reported that the mean number of working hours in a certain department is 42 hours per week. This would have been calculated as the total number of hours worked by all the personnel divided by the number of personnel.

The mean rating of the nurses from the liver infection survey is therefore calculated as follows:

$$\text{Mean} = \frac{275}{50} = 5.5$$

The median

The median is the point on a scale that has an equal number of scores above and below it. This is known as the 50th percentile and is used to describe 'typical' performance. To obtain the median, the scores should be arranged in ascending numerical order. If there is an even number of scores, place the median midway between the (N/2) score and the (N/2) + 1 score. If there is an odd number of scores, place the median at the score that is the (N + 1)/2 from the bottom.

For example, five coping styles were ranked for in order of increasing patient comfort.

CS1	3
CS2	6
CS3	12
CS4	13
CS5	19

The median score is 12 and the median coping style is therefore CS3. Results could then be reported in terms of those coping styles that had higher and lower levels of comfort than the median.

Note how the median does not take into account extreme scores so that if the coping styles were actually rated as:

CS1	3
CS2	6
CS3	12
CS4	13
CS5	2,300

The median score would still be 12. Because of this, the median is often used for reporting the typical score of an ordinal or ranked scale or for reporting the central tendency of a skewed distribution.

Note that the cumulative distribution frequency can be used to compute the median. The median score can be calculated as being the score that is at the 50th percentile.

The mode

The mode is a score (or a point on the score scale) that has a higher frequency than other scores in that distribution. It describes the prevailing characteristic of the majority of Respondents *(for example, the most popular career amongst one cohort of doctors was General Practice)*. In general, the mode is not widely used because it can fluctuate from sample to sample and is not suitable for further statistical computation.

Variation: range, variance and standard deviation

When reporting an average, the Researcher should always report the spread or dispersion of the scores (i.e. the range or variation). Knowledge of the variability in the data is crucial since it tells the Researcher how homogeneous the data are and, therefore, how representative they are of the measure of central tendency. For example, consider again the fictitious ratings made by the nurses of their likelihood of catching an infection when working in a liver transplant ward. If the ratings were a lot more varied (i.e. the scores were dispersed across the whole rating scale), then it would be hard to draw conclusions about the mean score. However, if most nurses provided about the same rating, then that same mean would be much more representative of the data. Consequently the variability in the data is as important an index to report as the measure of central tendency.

The range

This is expressed as the spread between the lowest and the highest score. Variation in ranked data is best represented by range only. *For example, during 1995 the average number of hours worked each week ranged between 35 and 65 for the staff of a certain department. Or, to continue with the nurse data example, it can be seen that the maximum score was 9 and the minimum score was 1. The range is therefore 8.*

The range is, however, a very unstable index of variability because it is based simply on two scores – the highest and the lowest – and ignores the variability in the scores between these two extremes. Therefore, this measure of variability is rarely used on its own and is more likely to be used in conjunction with some other measure of variation.

The interquartile range measures the range of the middle 50% of the data and is easily measured from the cumulative frequency distribution. The interquartile range is the difference between the scores equivalent to the 25th percentile and the 75th percentile. Since this index is a measure based on the middle 50% of the data, it is considerably more stable than the range.

Variance and standard deviation

Like the range, these two closely related terms describe the spread of the scores but, unlike the range, the variance and the standard deviation measure variation inherent in all the data. These measures are based on a score's distance from the mean. The variance and the standard deviation can be computed only from continuous data.

The following example shows why reporting the standard deviation is important. The mean job satisfaction of one group of community health professionals compared to another was the same. However, the standard deviation in Group A was larger than in Group B, indicating that there was more variation in their reported job satisfaction. Such a result suggests that there are differences between the groups and that our trust in the mean score of Group A should be less than our trust in the mean score of Group B.

To calculate the standard deviation, follow a four-stage process.

1. Calculate the difference between each number and the mean score:

   $x = (X - \bar{x})$

2. Square these values of x.
3. Add up all these 'squared deviations from the mean' and then divide by the number of scores. This gives a measure of the variance:

$$VAR = \frac{\Sigma x^2}{N}$$

where Σx = all the individual scores and N is the number of scores.
4. Take the square root of the variance to give the standard deviation.

The following simple example explains how the standard deviation is calculated:

Score	$\bar{x}$	$x = X - \bar{x}$ (Step 1)	$x^2 = (X - \bar{x})^2$ (Step 2)
3	4	−1	1
4	4	0	0
6	4	2	4
4	4	0	0
3	4	−1	1
		$\Sigma x = 0$	$\Sigma x^2 = 6$

(Step 3) VAR = 6/5 = 1.2
(Step 4) SD = $\sqrt{1.2}$ = 1.1

Most Researchers will, as a matter of course, report the standard deviation of the data along with the mean. What does the standard deviation represent?

(a) the standard deviation is an index of the variability of the data. The distribution that has a lower standard deviation is more homogeneous than a distribution with a larger standard deviation.

(b) when a standard deviation from a normal distribution (bell-shaped) is found, it is possible to draw further conclusions about the data from knowledge of this one statistic alone. Here a fixed percentage of cases fall within certain distances from the mean:

68% of cases fall within one standard deviation of the mean
95% of cases fall within 1.96 standard deviations from the mean (often rounded to 2).

If a distribution follows a normal curve, this can be a useful way of classifying how extreme a certain score is. *For example, a survey was administered to determine the popularity of a local hospital in the community. A total of 100 Respondents replied and the data followed a normal distribution. The mean score on a 10-point scale was 4 and the standard deviation was therefore 2. Sixty-eight per cent (68%) of Respondents therefore reported their ratings as between 2 and 6 (i.e. one standard deviation above and below the mean) and 95% of Respondents reported their ratings as between 0.08 and 7.92 (i.e. 1.96 standard deviations above and below the mean). Any ratings below .08 or above 7.92 were only made by 5% of the Respondents (i.e. 5 people).*

The interested reader may like to check that the standard deviation of the nurses' perception of risk when working in a liver transplant ward is 1.96 and the variance is 3.85.

Contingency tables and correlations

Sometimes the Researcher is interested in finding relationships between variables instead of just describing a single variable.

Correlations show relationships between groups:

(a) Contingency tables are used with nominal data or ordinal data that consist of just a few categories
(b) Pearson product-moment correlations are used to establish relationships between two sets of continuous data (from interval and ratio scales). Although this statement is not strictly true of attitude rating scales, many Researchers include most of the latter types of scale in this category.
(c) Spearman rank-order correlations are used with categorical data (from ordinal scales).

Contingency tables

Contingency tables are simply cross-tabulations of frequency distributions. Refer back to the frequency distribution of the nurse data presented in Table 3. If the Researcher believed there were sex differences in the ratings then it would be further possible to classify the ratings according to whether or not the data were provided by male or female nurses. The reclassification of the raw data is shown in Table 4. A two-way frequency distribution is now calculated to determine if sex has an effect on the nurses' perception of risk (Table 5). This simple procedure allows the Researcher to see that male nurses tend to provide lower ratings of risk than female nurses.

Table 4. Ratings by nurses classified according to their sex

		Male nurses			Ratings made by		Female nurses		
5	4	5	5	3	7	4	4	7	9
5	3	5	5	4	7	5	6	8	2
6	5	6	1	5	7	8	5	5	7
7	7	7	2	4	8	8	5	4	6
5	2	8	4	5	9	9	8	3	6

Table 5. Contingency table of sex/ratings of risk relationship

Ratings	Male nurses	Female nurses	Total sample of nurses
1	1 4% of males	–	1 2% of sample
2	2 8% of males	1 4% of females	3 6% of sample
3	2 8% of males	1 4% of females	3 6% of sample
4	4 16% of males	3 12% of females	7 14% of sample
5	10 40% of males	4 16% of females	14 28% of sample
6	2 8% of males	3 12% of females	5 10% of sample
7	3 12% of males	5 20% of females	8 16% of sample
8	1 4% of males	5 20% of females	6 12% of sample
9	–	3 12% of females	3 6% of sample
Column Total	25 50% of sample	25 50% of sample	50 100% of sample

Correlations

The most widely used measure of the relationship between two variables is the correlation. The main question asked is: How much are two variables related to each other? For example, is wound recovery related to the amount of time the wound is left open, or is career success related to ambition?

The degree of relationship between two variables can be shown graphically by means of a scatter-plot or by calculation as one of two forms of the correlation coefficient.

The scatter-plot is easily calculated using the following technique. The two variables are classified according to the subject. Fictitious data relating anxiety to length of stay in hospital after childbirth for each of 10 subjects is shown in Table 6. The anxiety scale was measured on a 1–5 rating scale where 5 indicated a highly anxious individual. This scale is plotted on the Y axis (the vertical) of the graph and the length of stay in hospital variable is plotted on the X axis (the horizontal).

Table 6. Data used in the construction of a scatter-plot

Subject	Anxiety	Length of stay in hospital (days) after childbirth
	Y	X
1	4	4
2	2	1
3	4	5
4	1	1
5	3	3
6	1	2
7	5	5
8	3	2
9	1	2
10	4	4

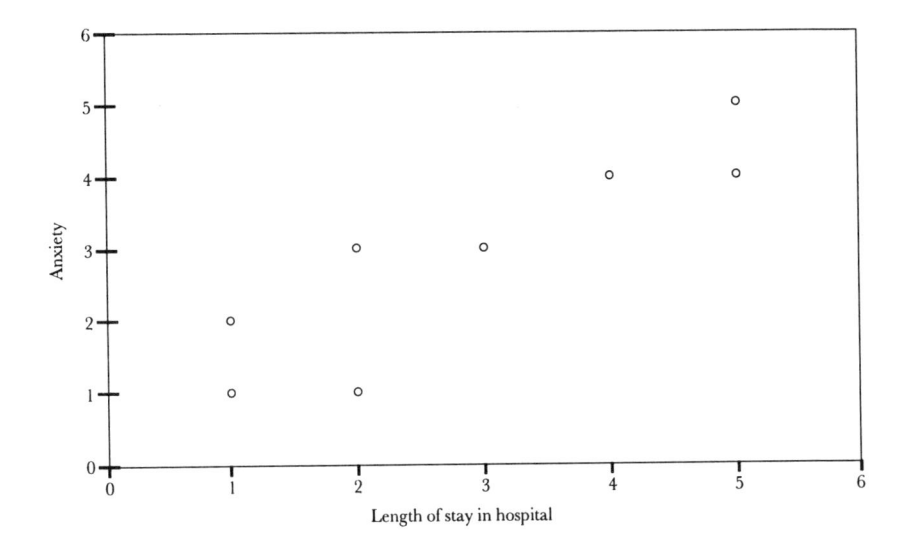

Figure 5. Scatter-plot of anxiety vs. length of stay in hospital.

The scatter-plot shown in Figure 5 describes a positive relationship between the two variables because the direction of the slope is from bottom left to top right. As anxiety increases, so does the length of stay in the hospital. It can be seen that the magnitude of the relationship is quite strong because low scorers on one scale tend to be low scorers on the other scale, and high scorers on one scale tend to be high scorers on the other scale. The closer the scatter-plot resembles a straight line through the points, the stronger the relationship.

A negative relationship would have been described if an increase in one variable was related to a decrease in the other. For example, an increase in exercise is likely to lead to a decrease in coronary heart disease in later life. If this relationship were plotted, the negative relationship would be shown as a series of points from bottom right to top left.

Figure 6 provides a graphical representation of different types of relationship between two variables.

Correlation coefficients provide a summary index of the relationship between two variables. Values range from +1 (perfect positive correlation) to −1 (perfect negative correlation). A correlation of 0 indicates that there is no relationship between the variables. The higher the correlation (whether it is negative or positive), the stronger the relationship.

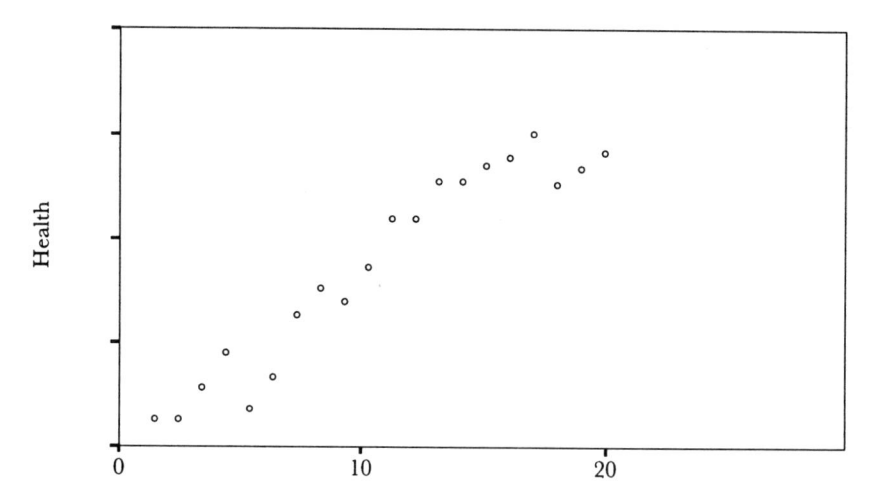

(1) Scatter-plot showing a positive relationship between two variables. The two variables have a high positive correlation suggesting that good health is related to high social class and poor health is related to low social class.

Figure 6a. Various possible relationships between two variables.

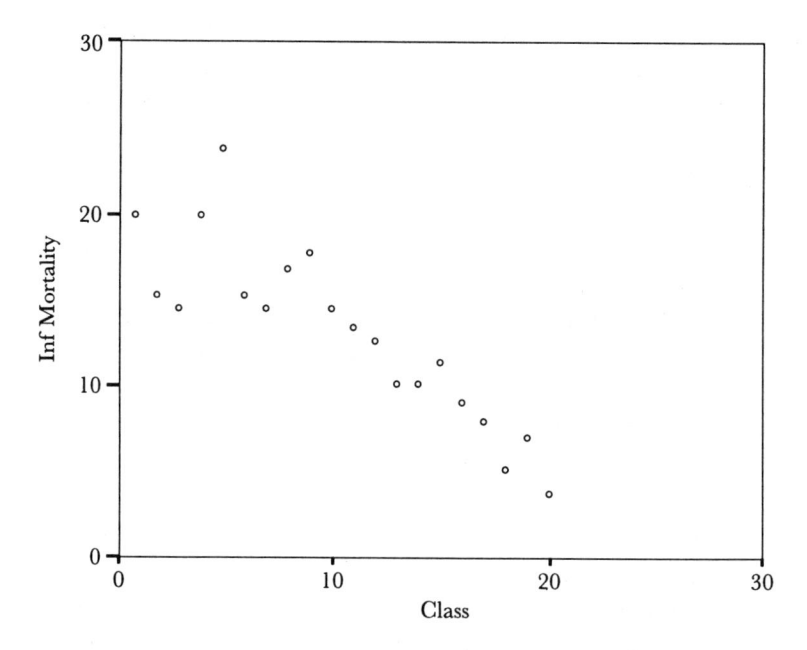

(2) Scatter-plot showing a high negative relationship between two variables. Here they have a high negative correlation –i.e. the plot suggests that infant mortality is higher when social class is lower.

Figure 6b. Various possible relationships between two variables.

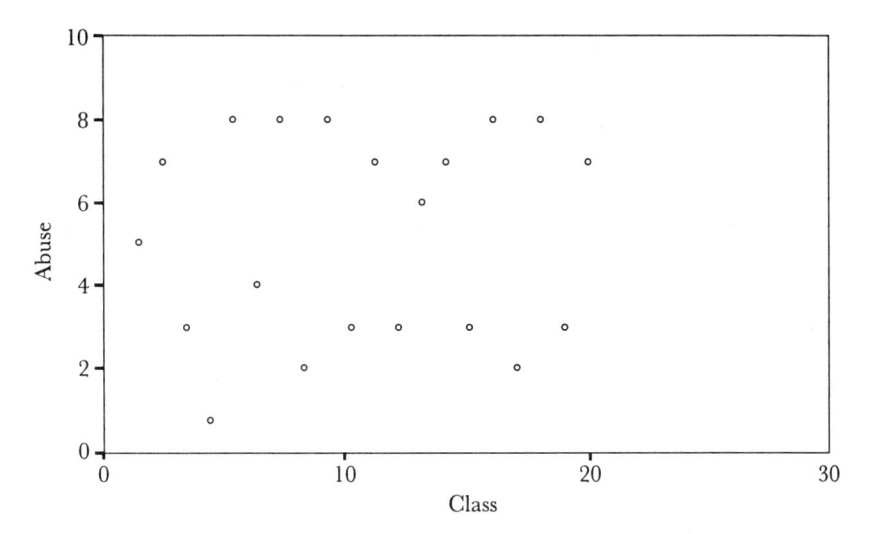

Analysing data from surveys 171

[scatter plot of Abuse (y-axis, 0–10) vs Class (x-axis, 0–30)]

(3) Scatter-plot showing no relationship between two variables. Here the correlation approximates zero with the indication that levels of abuse are not related to social class.

Figure 6c. Various possible relationships between two variables.

When trying to determine the meaning of a correlation, it should be noted that correlations cannot be used to establish causation. *For example, a reasonably strong correlation may be reported between vitamin intake and IQ. This is an interesting observation but it does not necessarily mean that vitamin intake* causes *an increase in IQ. This might be the case but equally it may be that generally brighter people tend to supplement their diets with vitamins or that some third factor (such as early learning environment) may cause both an increase in vitamin consumption and IQ.*

It should also be noted that correlations close to +1 or −1 are extremely rare in survey or questionnaire research. Quite often a Researcher would believe a relationship to be reasonably strong (i.e. meaningful) if it were over 0.3. Researchers are also often interested in assessing whether or not the correlation is significantly different from zero. This is easily done by looking at statistical tables developed for this purpose. Note that there are N −2 degrees of freedom where N is the number of subjects.

The most widely used index to express the relationship between two interval or ratio scales is Pearson's product-moment correlation coefficient (r). Spearman's rank correlation (rho) is suitable for assessing the degree of relationship between two ranked variables. First, determine the rank order of each variable and second, perform a Pearson product-moment correlation on the rank order. There are many other types of correlation available if the data suggest that Pearson's r or Spearman's rho are inappropriate.

Whereas we have provided example calculations up to this point, this is where we draw a line. Calculation of the correlation coefficient is straightforward but laborious. In fact, it is rarely done by hand in applied research because it is almost always calculated by computer.

Comparisons

The purpose of this section is to alert the Researcher to the possibilities of further analysis. Many Researchers will not feel the need to report the results of their survey in a more complex form than has already been discussed. In fact, as already noted, many Researchers believe that simple percentages represent the perfect level of analysis! If a Researcher wishes to do comparisons or more complex and sophisticated statistics then advanced texts should be studied, or an expert consulted. It is easy to enter the data in a statistics software package and ask the package to perform the analysis. However, unless the input, technique and output are clearly understood, the chances of error are too high for us to recommend that an inexperienced Researcher try them. The authors believe that best practice in performing relatively complex statistics is to have a far clearer understanding of them than this text is designed to provide. We are thus unwilling to go halfway, and therefore limit ourselves to a brief explanation of further statistical methods.

The following statistics are widely used to make comparisons:

(a) The Mann-Whitney U test is used to compare two independent groups with data from nominal responses
(b) The chi-square is used to identify associations between nominal data
(c) The t-test enables a comparison to be made of the average views of two groups and determines the probability of a difference between them being real and not due to chance. Data should be continuous, and there should be at least 20 cases per group to compare. Confidence intervals are commonly used as alternatives to t-tests. *For example, an independent t-test was used to report a significant difference between the average job satisfaction scores of female nurses and male nurses. It was found that on average female nurses were less satisfied than male nurses.*

(d) An analysis of variance (ANOVA) permits two or more groups to be compared at the same time.
(e) To measure trends (i.e. changes over a period of time for the same group of individuals) the Researcher should employ special forms of t-tests and ANOVAs: either a paired t-test to measure change in a single group between two time periods or a repeated measure ANOVA to measure changes in one or more groups between two or more time periods.

Regression

Regression is widely used by professionals to develop a model that can be used to make predictions. A Researcher may wish to predict a variable from one or more other variables. Thus on the basis of known data on a variable, a prediction can be made about some other variable.

For example, three variables may be measured in a survey: (a) a measure of obesity; (b) amount of food eaten on average in a day in calories; (c) amount of time spent exercising on average in a day.

The Researcher could determine the optimal model for predicting obesity from intake of calories and time spent exercising by regressing obesity against food intake and time spent exercising. Regression would determine the equation of this model. Once the equation is known, it is possible to use it in prediction of obesity for new subjects based on the information given.

The following points will help the Researcher to understand the principles used in regression:

(a) Linear regression is used to predict one variable (the dependent variable) from another (the independent variable), whereas multiple linear regression is used to predict one variable from several independent variables.
(b) In linear regression, the higher the correlation between a dependent variable and an independent variable, the more accurate is the prediction. A perfect correlation (either +1 or −1) between the dependent and independent variable would result in an equation that could provide a perfect prediction.
(c) In multiple regression, the strength of the relationship between dependent and independent variables is related to the correlation between each independent variable and the dependent variables, and to the correlations between the dependent variables. Since

the addition of more independent variables inevitably tends to lead to higher correlations between them, there is a decreasing return from adding more and more variables into the equation.
(d) Linear regression works by determining the equation of the line which minimizes the error sums of squares.
(e) The basic formula that is fitted for linear regression is:

$$Y = a + bX$$

where Y is the dependent variable, X is a independent variable, a is the constant and b is the regression weight (or gradient of the regression line)

and the basic formula for multiple regression is

$$Y = a + b_1X_1 + b_2X_2 + \ldots + b_kX_k$$

for k independent variables.
(f) r is used to show the strength of the prediction for linear multiple regression; R is used to show the strength of the relationship in multiple regression. R is always positive so does not show the direction of the relationship (R cannot show the direction of the relationship because some independent variables may show a positive relationship and others a negative relationship).
(g) R^2 is a direct measure of the amount of variability explained in the dependent variable by the independent variables.
(h) The significance of each regression weight provides information about the significance of each independent variable. A t-test determines if the regression weight is significantly different from zero.
(i) Multiple regression provides little information in its most simple form about the relative contribution of each independent variable because the regression weight depends upon the correlation of that independent variable with other independent variables as well as with the dependent variable. In other words, if two independent variables are highly correlated with each other and yet both are very important, only one of them will be significant in the multiple regression equation.
(j) Stepwise multiple regression is often used to determine which of many independent variables are useful in predicting a dependent

variable. When used, the independent variables are entered into the equation in order of their predictive power until there is no improvement in R^2.

Factor analysis

Factor analysis is used to summarize a large set of variables (such as items in a survey or scales in a survey) into a smaller, more understandable set. Thus factor analysis can be used to determine or to confirm (1) that certain items within a questionnaire are related enough to each other to form a single dimension or (2) that scales are related enough to each other to become higher order factors (e.g. extroversion can be thought of as a combination of second-order factors of sociability and impulsiveness).

We can demonstrate factor analysis at two different levels. First, factor analysis can be used to determine the factor structure of items in a questionnaire or survey. For example, the following results could have been obtained from a factor analysis of a personality questionnaire. We show the six items of the questionnaire down the left-hand side of the page, and the correlation (the factor loading) between each item and the first two theoretical factors on the right-hand side. Note how each item has a high correlation with one factor but not the other. We say that the factor with the highest meaningful correlation is the factor that the item loads on. Thus items 1, 2 and 3 load on factor I and items 4, 5, and 6 load on factor II. The results also tells us that factor I explains 40% of the variation in the data matrix and factor II explains 20%. Other factors not shown explain the remaining 40% of the variation.

	I 40%	II 20%
I have lots of friends	**0.85**	0.01
I like going to parties	**0.86**	0.02
I am not fond of reading	**0.76**	0.01
I get anxious when things go wrong	0.02	**0.91**
I am scared of snakes	0.04	**0.88**
My mood changes quickly	0.10	**0.79**

The Researcher must then name factor I and factor II. In this case the most obvious name for factor I is Extroversion and the most obvious name for factor II is Neuroticism. However Sociability and Anxiety or other similar labels could have been chosen and just as easily justified by the Researcher.

Second, factor analysis can be used to identify higher factor structure to scales that have been derived from a questionnaire or survey. Thus factor analysis of six personality scales could have produced the following results:

	I 50%	II 30%
Ambition	**0.74**	0.01
Sociability	**0.67**	0.23
Assertiveness	**0.78**	0.15
Anxiety	0.21	**0.67**
Guilt	0.32	**0.45**
Inferiority	0.45	**0.78**

The Researcher would examine this factor loading matrix to determine the underlying factor structure to the six variables. Again, the Researcher would probably decide that the three first scales would load on a higher order factor labelled Extroversion and the last three scales would load on a factor called Neuroticism.

These examples are made up to provide a simple introduction to the subject, but real-life factor analysis is less simple and requires much greater skills of interpretation. One of the ways to simplify these factor loading matrices is to show only factor loadings above a certain level. Box 20 provides a relatively simple real-life example of one of the ways of making factor analysis comprehensible.

Box 20

Factor Loading for the Attitudes to Phobia Questionnaire

	Factor			
	1	2	3	4
1. Phobias always originate with early childhood experiences.	.42			
2. People with phobias are rather dependent, clinging sort of people.	.85			

Analysing data from surveys

3. People with phobias tend to be timid, shy
   and highly introverted people. .82
4. Women are more likely than men to
   develop phobias. .42
5. We can inherit phobias from the genes
   which we get from our parents. .70
6. Our genes affect our personality and can
   indirectly affect the likelihood of our .77
   developing a phobia.
7. Phobias are caused by a chemical .68
   imbalance in the brain.
8. Phobias nearly always develop after a
   frightening or traumatic event.
9. People often learn their phobias from their
   parents or close family when they are young. .44
10. Our cultural background can affect the
    likelihood of development of a phobia. .82
11. Even watching certain films (e.g. Jaws)
    can make someone phobic. .82
12. Nearly everyone has some sort of phobia. .41
13. We can develop a phobia to absolutely
    any object or situation. .74
14. Some phobias develop because we
    associate non-traumatic objects with
    traumatic ones (e.g. become phobic .79
    about roses because you were stung by
    a bee while picking them).
15. People become phobic about certain
    things (snakes and heights) because in doing
    so they increase their chances of survival.
16. Phobias which develop after just one .42
    frightening experience can last for life.
17. Once a person has developed a fear it
    can easily generalize to similar objects (fear .62
    of rats leads to fear of all furry objects).

(Adapted from Furnham, 1995)

To make the table easier to understand we include only the highest factor loadings of each item and only those greater than 0.4. Varimax rotation was used and here the first four factors are shown.

(contd)

> This provides a list of the items on each factor that are highly interrelated and therefore should comprise a single scale. This way of reducing the factor loading matrix provides a simple means of interpreting a matrix of correlations that would otherwise be completely uninterpretable (and this is just a short questionnaire!). In the original study, Factor 1 was labelled 'Personality' because the items refer to individual differences of the aetiology of phobia; Factor 2 was labelled 'Physical' because items concerned genetic or biochemical determinants of phobia; Factor 3 was labelled 'observational learning' because the items imply that phobias could be learned by observing phobic responses; Factor 4 was labelled 'behavioural pairing' because the items suggested that associative learning was a major cause.

Researchers and Clients need to understand the pros and cons associated with factor analysis. The pros are that it is a very powerful technique that works and really appears to extract a useful and meaningful structure from a set of data; the cons are that the interpretation of factor analysis is very subjective and that multiple and different solutions can be found that are mathematically equivalent. It is, therefore, up to the Researcher to choose the best solution (i.e. how to extract factors, how many factors to extract, and how to rotate the factors as discussed in Boxes 21 and 22). All this can lead to misguided enthusiasm about a solution that has little practical relevance. By this we mean that factor analysis may extract variables that only exist mathematically, and have much less of a basis in the real world. Thus psychologists still debate whether there are 3, 5, 16 or another set of factors that describe human personality, because a multitude of factor analyses on multiple data sets seem to produce results which cannot discriminate between them. Again, as in much of this section, our message is that factor analysis may be easily done by computer but the interpretation of the results should only be undertaken by a skilled practitioner who understands the theory and practice of factor analysis.

Analysing data from surveys

Box 21

How many factors to extract?

The first hurdle for the factor analyst to overcome is the question of how many factors to extract from the factor analysis. Researchers have found that rotation of too few factors or too many factors tends to produce too broad or too narrow factors respectively.

The default solution with many software packages is to rotate factors with eigenvalues greater than one. Eigenvalues tell us the amount of variance that each factor explains; if the eigenvalue is above one, then it is explaining more than each of the original items.

However, there is now reasonable agreement amongst factor analysts that Cattell's scree slope provides the best available solution. With this method, the eigenvalues are plotted against the extracted factors, and the number of factors to be rotated is shown by the change in slope of the resultant line. An example scree slope is shown in Figure 7 and it can be seen that four factors would be extracted.

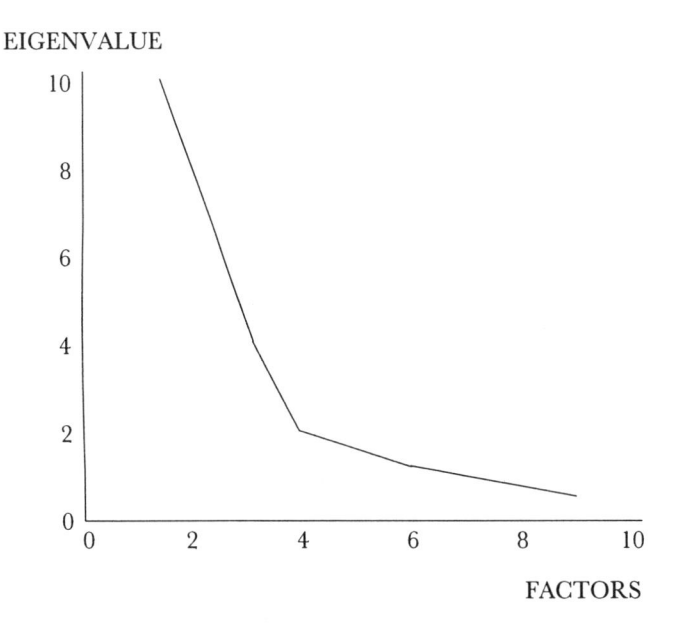

Figure 7. Example Scree Slope.

> **Box 22**
>
> **What is factor rotation?**
>
> Once it has been determined how many factors there are in the factor analytical solution, a rotation must be performed. The purpose of rotation is to identify a mathematical solution that provides the most readily interpretable factor loading matrix. Although there are many ways of carrying out a rotation, we will only discuss the results obtained from the varimax method, which is the one most widely used. Varimax rotation produces a readily understandable set of orthogonal factors. In other words, the factors that are produced tend to have high or low (not medium) correlations with the original items, and the factors are uncorrelated with each other.

Cronbach's Alpha

Cronbach's Alpha is often quoted as a measure of the internal consistency of the items that are thought to comprise a certain content area or scale within a survey or questionnaire. Internal consistency is used as a measure of how similar the items are to each other. It is a measure of the integrity or consistency of the scale. Cronbach's Alpha should be above 0.7 for most professionally constructed scales. Low figures indicate that the items have little similarity with each other. Sometimes figures of over 0.85 indicate tautology, which can therefore also be a poor indicator of scale quality owing to redundant items having been included in the scale. For the statistically minded, Cronbach's Alpha is the average of all the split-half reliabilities that can be computed.

Computation of the statistics

All survey data should be analysed by computer. For this reason we are not discussing the equations for computing the statistics here. It is possible to analyse data using statistics packages (e.g. SPSS and MINITAB), spreadsheets (e.g. EXCEL), or specialized survey analysis packages that appear on the market from time to time. Statistics packages are preferable but more complex. Spreadsheets are powerful tools, and potentially advantageous for the inexperienced because they can do so much in a short time. However, this advantage is something of a two-edged sword as it makes the user vulnerable to fundamental errors that can undermine the whole analysis.

Statistical significance

Having performed a survey, perhaps one that compares the behaviour or attitudes of two groups, it is necessary to evaluate the significance of the results and determine whether any observed differences between the groups are due to chance alone. Anything that is unlikely to happen by chance is termed statistically significant. Generally a probability (p-value) of less than 5% ($p < 0.05$) is regarded as significant. A Researcher should always quote levels of significance when performing a statistical test.

Summary

In this chapter we have described the methods usually applied in the analysis of data from surveys and questionnaires. In general, we have advised Researchers to use statistical methods of analysis that they feel competent to use and that will be suitable for their audience. For many Researchers this will mean producing percentages, means and standard deviations. The reality is that it is rare for a Client to ask for analyses more complex than this.

Nevertheless, most survey data can be analysed with more sophisticated techniques (e.g. tests of significance, multiple regression and factor analysis). Although these generally require a much greater level of expertise, they have excellent potential as a means of answering more in-depth questions about the data. Inexperienced Researchers will be out of their depth when trying to use them and there is a great danger of making elementary mistakes that undermine the whole analysis.

Part 6:
The report

Chapter 12
Presenting the survey results

Introduction

Results of a survey are usually presented in a formal report submitted by the Researcher to the Client (and/or others). Usually the survey results are presented as tables, graphs and pictures together with appropriate explanations and descriptions. Apart from the actual results, which should also be verbally described, the Researcher must include a full description of the survey.

The contents of a written report

Before starting to write the report, the Researcher should make a judgement on its technical level, and the amount of detail required for the expected readership. For example, an academic report should be comprehensive and properly referenced. A more commercial report should be just as thoroughly researched, but may need to be short and to the point. Moreover, there is no point in using sophisticated statistics and survey jargon that the readers will not be able to understand because they are not familiar with the subject. Similarly, a simple report that does not include a suitable statistic for a 'clever' audience may easily be criticized. Wise Researchers who believe in 'best practice' will know their audience well.

A report should consist of the following:

(a) An abstract: This should be approximately 150–200 words in length, and should include:
   – The objective

- The method employed
- The sample size and response rate
- Findings
- Cautions

(b) A management summary. This is an extended version of the abstract. It can be up to three pages in length and may include key tables.
(c) A table of contents. This should list all major sections with page numbers.
(d) A list of tables and figures. Full titles and page numbers should be given.
(e) A glossary of terms. This should include all technical terms and special abbreviations.
(f) Purposes. These give the survey's objectives, i.e. its reasons and expectations and hypotheses to be tested.
(g) Method. This should describe what the Researcher did and should include the following:
- Type of survey
- Questions asked (examples or whole survey)
- Survey logistics (personnel involved)
- Survey constructions.
- Sampling and response rate
- Design (cross-sectional, etc.)
(h) Findings. These are results of the survey properly analysed and presented in an easy to understand format.
(i) Discussion. This should connect the findings to the objectives, and point out any unexpected results.

Selection of presentational material

Criteria for selecting tables, graphs, etc., are given below:

(a) Accuracy: A major objective should be to present the results accurately, simply and informatively.
(b) Convention or expectations. The Client may expect greater detail and more in-depth information of tables, or simple easy-to-understand graphs.
(c) Ability and resources: Use computers and electronic printers to substantially reduce the cost and effort of producing tables and graphs.

Using tables

Tables in survey reports are used to describe Respondents and their environment, show relationships, and describe changes and combinations of relationships and changes. Their contents include the number of Respondents, the groups being compared, the times for observing change and the results of the survey.

To prepare tables the Researcher should:

(a) Set a limit on the number of columns and rows required to avoid including so much information that the table becomes unreadable.
(b) Have a title that summarizes the purpose and contents of the table.
(c) Make the source of the data immediately obvious; it should be given at the foot of the table.
(d) Define new terms in footnotes.
(e) Place additional information after the table in the main body of the report.
(f) Select a particular table format and adhere to it consistently, e.g. use of capitals in captions and labels.
(g) Present the data in a logical order.
(h) Ensure the sample size is included and differentiate between numbers and percentages.

Using pie diagrams

Pie diagrams are useful in illustrating the proportion of each response category to the whole. With modern computer software they are easy to design, complete with titles, labels and percentage contribution. In general, no more than six sectors should be shown in any one pie. It is important to bear in mind that pie diagrams are excellent means of conveying a small amount of information but are too large for many to be included in most survey reports. Therefore the Researcher must be very selective in the use of these diagrams.

Using bar graphs

Bar graphs are widely used to display comparative data, generally as a function of some other parameter, such as time. Once again, they can easily be drawn up with a computer and are good at displaying information, but they are also large. The Researcher needs to convey only the most important information with this technique.

Using line graphs

Line graphs permit the comparison of groups, the showing of trends and the identification of patterns.

Rules for preparing graphs:

(a) The Y (vertical) and X (horizontal) axes should be of about equal length and sensibly scaled. Do not show meaningless trends by exaggerating scales.
(b) Choose the variables on the X axis and Y axis carefully. Usually the X axis will be the variable that changes regularly (e.g. time and year), and the Y axis will be the variable that changes irregularly (e.g. pay, satisfaction, culture).
(c) Equal numeric differences should be represented by equal physical differences on all scales.
(d) As well as titles and labels, etc., keys to lines and symbols must be given.
(e) Keep the graph as simple as possible.

The Researcher needs to bear in mind the strengths of this graphical technique in comparison to the amount of space it uses within the report.

Pictures

Pictures will rarely be needed with survey data. However, they might prove useful in particular circumstances, (e.g. if the results showed a geographical spread, these could be annotated on a map of the area).

The oral presentation

Presenters should speak clearly and slowly, and avoid long, convoluted sentences. However, it is not possible to cover as many points as would be possible in a written report, because listeners simply do not have sufficient time to grasp all the detailed information. Therefore, it is necessary to restrict the talk to the most important aspects only. These should be introduced at the beginning, amplified during the main part of the presentation, and referred to again at the close.

Useful aids to oral presentation of survey material are:

(a) Handouts: These may consist of tables, graphs or summaries. The audience's attention should be drawn to these at the start of the talk.
(b) Transparencies: These should be in large, bold type and limited to short, simple sentences, with perhaps only six lines per sheet. Graphs and tables may also be shown, but they must be kept simple if people at the back of the audience are to be able to read them.
(c) Slides: These are an excellent way of presenting graphs, tables and pictures. Once again, simplicity is most important.

Software packages are also increasingly being used to enhance the quality of transparencies, slides and audio productions. The presenter will often use a combination of computer and projector to add an audiovisual or multimedia experience to a presentation.

During a presentation, a Researcher may have to overcome objections to the use of surveys. Among the most common and sensible objections voiced at presentations are that:

(a) Many surveys are potentially biased or faked. Careful design and honest reporting of results minimizes this objection. Being well read and having done background research will give the Researcher the broad perspective to overcome intelligent criticism.
(b) Surveys are unreliable because temporary factors (e.g. anxiety, boredom weariness, a headache, etc.) cause Respondents to give different answers on different occasions. As a general rule, this factor makes only a small difference.
(c) Surveys are invalid, i.e. they do not measure what they say they are measuring and scores do not predict behaviour over time. For poorly designed surveys this is a real problem because conclusions are drawn which are simply not correct. Well designed and executed surveys are likely to be much more valid.
(d) Respondents have to be sufficiently literate and articulate to complete a survey. If your respondents may fall in this category, the surveys should be conducted by face-to-face interview.
(e) Surveys do not establish causal relationships between variables. There is some truth in the lack of causality and this interpretation

is often what the Researcher must add. Conclusions drawn must be reflected by the results.

(f) Surveys are incapable of getting at meaningful aspects of social behaviour because Respondents have wills, goals, memories and motivation. Often, however, this is exactly what a survey directly sets out to measure. A Researcher is wise to remember that survey technique may be flawed but nevertheless it is the best that is available in many instances.

Summary

The Researcher should:

(a) Choose the appropriate way of showing the results to their best advantage and yet in an unbiased manner.
(b) Write the report in a clear, concise style.
(c) Include details about the method so that the Client can judge the quality of the survey.
(d) Prepare for oral presentations and be prepared to overcome criticism of the survey method.

Chapter 13
Evaluating reports

Introduction

Knowing what to look for when evaluating research for potential inclusion in the literature review or knowing what to look for when evaluating a Researcher's work is one of the most important skills that those sponsoring research, or involved in research, can acquire. It is only through the critical appraisal of work that it can be put into proper context and its relevance and appropriateness understood. Couchman and Dawson (1990) suggest that the reader should be something of a detective. There will be clues and twists in the plot that will need to be followed. Finally the reader will have to decide if the author is justified in coming up with the conclusions that have been drawn on the evidence that has been presented. Couchman and Dawson suggest that a reader should ask these key questions:

(a) What was the study about?
(b) Why was it done?
(c) How was it done?
(d) Are the findings justified, explained and relevant?

The structure of reports

Clients expect a report to have a simple and comprehensible structure. All formal survey reports should describe:

(a) What the principal research question was.

(b) Why this needs to be investigated (and perhaps what previous research has been conducted in this area).
(c) What the research method was.
(d) What the results are.
(e) What conclusions can be drawn.

Of course not all research is formally reported and in such cases the format can vary. It may be that reports written for administrators are shortened so that just the results and conclusions are presented. Equally a report written for a popular 'professional' magazine such as *Nursing Times*, *Social Work Today*, or *The Health Visitor* may be brief and give very little detail about anything but the most important introductory points, the principal results and the key conclusions. These popular articles tend to skip over the details because they are seen as too tedious for the typical reader. As a result of this, it will be difficult to judge the quality of the work from the article; in general the reader is expected to believe in the validity of the work on the basis of the writer's authority.

Assessing the quality of reports

When reading a report and assessing the quality of the research, the following steps can be followed:

(a) Read the summary/abstract
(b) Look at the introduction to see what the Researcher was doing and why the work was done.
(c) Have a brief look at the major results to gain an overview of what the Researcher claims to have found.
(d) Read the conclusions to see what the Researcher thinks the results mean.
(e) Now the reader should look deeper below the surface of the research report to assess the quality of the evidence and arguments as well as to understand the wider implications of the work.

The first step must be to determine if the research has validity. Are the conclusions justified on the basis of the evidence that has been presented? It may be, for example, that there are alternative, just as plausible, conclusions that can be drawn from the evidence. Perhaps there are also alternative theories that fit the evidence but were not tested by the data. Is it possible that important variables that could influence the results were not measured? Are the variables reliable (i.e. consistent as opposed to being at the mercy of chance) and are the measures valid (i.e. measuring what they are supposed to be measuring). See Box 23 for a list of some of the ways the reader can be critical about reports. See Box 24 for a list of some of the ways the reader can be fooled into thinking there is more to a report than there actually is.

Box 23

Maxims for distinguishing a scientific report from the non-scientific

Marks and Kammann (1980) report various maxims for determining the basis of whether or not a report is best practice (i.e. produced scientifically) or of dubious value (i.e. not produced scientifically):

1. Ask the Researcher exactly what the theory predicts.
2. Find out from the Researcher how the evidence can be disproved.
3. Place the burden of proof with the Researcher. The Researcher should be able to substantiate belief in the theory.
4. How else could the evidence produced by the Researcher be explained? The Researcher may not have explored alternative possibilities.
5. Has evidence that could disprove the theory been omitted from the report. Sometimes evidence in favour of a theory seems stronger than it really is because only 'positive' evidence is reported.
6. Do not believe anecdotal evidence or testimonials.
7. Question the source of the theory and the history of the theory. Question the completeness and the balance of the literature review.
8. Question the emotional attachment that the Researcher has to the theory and the reported work. The more a Researcher becomes involved with a particular topic, the greater the possibility that scientific objectivity will be replaced by personal

(contd)

bias. For example, Researchers who are critical of the theory may well be classified as 'nasty' or 'stupid' so that their arguments can be rejected out of hand. It is also possible that the Researcher will turn against a critical Client accusing him of various underhand tactics. All of these arguments are fallacious, and it is important not only to recognize them, but to avoid them in your own work. 'The object is to learn, not to win' (Marks and Kamman, 1980, p.226).

Box 24

The art of illusory writing: Astrology and Graphology

Astrology and graphology are firmly enshrined within our culture. Although many people are sceptical about their validity, the fact remains that vast numbers of people are believers. These methods provide useful, 'fascinating' information perhaps in terms of a written report or as verbal feedback, but also claim to predict the future, thereby reducing anxieties and uncertainties about what will happen. Also, unlike other forms of therapy which require a psychological investment and/or behaviour change to obtain any benefit, in graphology one merely has to supply a written specimen, or in astrology the exact time and place of birth. There is much to gain and little to lose when visiting the astrologist or graphologist. As a result, a comfortable collaborative illusion of scientific validity emerges, formed between the buyer and seller of astrological readings and handwriting analyses.

There is another reason why people believe in graphology and astrology. This is the self-fulfilling prophecy. It seems likely that if a person is told 'as an Aries, you are particularly dynamic', this may lead that person to notice and subsequently recall selectively any or all instances of dynamic behaviour, however trivial, thus confirming the original report. The self-fulfilling prophecy may work on both a conceptual and a behavioural basis. Thus Aries people begin to include the trait of dynamism in their self-concept and may actually become a bit more active. The predictions of graphology and

> astrology may come true because accepting the predictions partly dictates that our behaviour will change appropriately.
>
> Beware the graphologist, the astrologer and *also* the conclusions derived from a poorly designed survey! The moral of all this is that the readers of any 'psychological report' can be impressed by the validity of a Researcher's 'psychological insights' or conclusions as long as they are vague, relevant, generally favourable, and personalized. Fortune tellers have exploited this fact for hundreds of years. Crystal balls and tarot cards have been replaced by simple pen and ink, but the principle remains the same. 'The fault of false belief is not in our stars, it is in ourselves.'

Further questions surround the notion of generalizability of the results of a survey. Most survey research is designed to draw conclusions that are relevant to the general population, or a specific part of that population. Almost always the research is not designed to inform only about the sample that has been involved in the research. (Contrast this with case reports about particular patients or members of staff, which are reports specifically written about a single individual). The problem of generalizability can be usefully illustrated with a couple of extreme examples. Conclusions from a sample drawn exclusively to explore the drinking habits of males are unlikely to represent women as well. Also conclusions drawn about one particular social class or race may not generalize into conclusions about the whole human race. A less extreme example may be the problems of generalizing from surveys that have been conducted by telephoning the home during the working day. Clearly the only people who can respond are those who are working at home, on holiday, sick or who are not in employment. Such respondents may not reflect the true diverse range of respondents. It is important for the Researcher to be aware of the extent that the work is generalisable to the wider population.

A final and important evaluation by the reader is the extent to which the Researcher has followed ethical guidelines. The basic minimum question for the reader to ask is: Was anyone harmed or overly inconvenienced by the research? Sapsford and Abbott (1992) phrase this well: Did the Researchers behave responsibly and leave the world no worse a place as a result of their investigation? The ethical point can be extended to determine whether the subjects benefited from their experience or, if they did not, was the research justified. Was the research commissioned for political reasons (for example as a tool to exploit staff) or was the survey fairly designed? Sapsford and Abbott point out that social research could be compared to an act of rape. A Researcher goes into a situation to conduct a survey, extracts exactly what he or she needs (such as information for the purpose of publication) and leaves the Respondents at best no worse off then they were when they started. The Respondents have been used to satisfy the needs of the Researcher. Whilst this is an extreme perspective, readers, Sponsors and Researchers need to be aware of the dangers of the negative way in which survey work can be portrayed.

Once these initial questions have been answered, the reader of the research report will want to return, hopefully with confidence in the report, to the paper's contents. Whilst taking into account the limitations of the research, the reader will want to become immersed in the substance of it. That is to say, the reader will be interested in understanding not only the major conclusion but the deeper components as well. Does it add knowledge? Does it inform or criticize present policy? Can it improve on the way things are presently done? Is the research a model that can be used to improve the design of further surveys?

Summary

Clients tend to be interested in obtaining answers to the following questions:

1. Is the research oriented towards the research questions?
2. Do the conclusions follow logically from what has been done?
3. Are there alternative conclusions to explain the results, which might undermine the conclusions that have been drawn?
4. Could the results be due to variables that were poorly measured, inaccurately measured or not measured at all? It is possible that the experimental design is seriously flawed?
5. Are the measurements valid and reliable?
6. Can the results be generalized to populations other than the sample that was used?
7. Was the research ethical? Was anyone emotionally damaged, hurt or inconvenienced by the research?

8. Does it seem as though the conclusions that were drawn were predetermined by the original question and design?
9. Are the results useful and relevant?

Chapter 14
Example reports together with introductory critiques

Finally, we reproduce three reports and present a critique on each. Read each report in turn and note down what you think is good and bad about them. Then compare your critiques with our own assessments of the reports (which we hope are reasonably unbiased)!

We gratefully acknowledge the permission to reproduce the reports from the publishers and note the source of the original publications:

1. Furnham A, Manning R (1997) Young people's theories of anorexia nervosa and obesity. Counselling Psychology Quarterly 10: 389–414. Published by Carfax Publishing Ltd, PO Box 25, Abingdon, Oxfordshire, OX14 3UE, United Kingdom.
2. Furnham A (1994) Explaining health and illness: lay perceptions on current and future health, the causes of illness and the nature of recovery. Social Science and Medicine 39: 715–25. Published by Elsevier Science, The Boulevard, Langford Lane, Kidlington, Oxford, OX5 1GB, United Kingdom.
3. Vincent C, Furnham A (1997) The perceived efficacy of complementary and orthodox medicine: a replication. Complementary Therapies in Medicine 5: 85–9. Published by Harcourt Brace, 24–8 Oval Road, London, NW1 7DX, United Kingdom.

Report 1

Young people's theories of anorexia nervosa and obesity by Adrian Furnham and Rachel Manning (Department of Psychology, University College London)

Abstract

One hundred and forty-seven participants completed a 108-item questionnaire (Furnham and Hume-Wright, 1992) that looked at their beliefs about the causes and cures of anorexia nervosa and obesity. The four parts of the questionnaire were individually factor analysed, and an interpretable factor structure emerged for each. While age and knowing someone with anorexia nervosa or obesity did not correlate with the factors obtained, sex, actual body size, estimated body size and having experience of an eating disorder were found to correlate significantly with a number of factors. Factors of cause and cure were not correlated regarding anorexia nervosa, but they were for obesity. Several correlations within cause and cure, across both disorders, were also significant. The implications of these findings, and how they relate to the theories described in the introduction, are considered in the discussion.

Introduction

The increase in both the scientific literature and popular press about eating disorders (especially anorexia nervosa) and obesity attests to increasing interest in this topic. Anorexia nervosa and obesity have many things in common. The prevalence of both is increasing, both are considered to have specific health risks, and many Researchers have made attempts to deal with the two together as eating disorders (Brownell and Foreyt, 1986; Bruch, 1973; Stock and Rothwell, 1982).

Anorexia nervosa is defined as a condition in which the patient has an abnormally low body weight, 25% below the original body weight, a disturbance of body image, an intense fear of becoming fat, no known medical illnesses leading to weight loss and other features such as amenorrhoea, suggesting a disordered physiology (Palmer, 1980). The disorder is sometimes also divided into primary and secondary anorexia. The sex ratio of female to male sufferers lies between 20:1 and 15:1 (Thompson, 1993). The higher incidence of anorexia nervosa in females may result from social factors affecting them (Hsu, 1983), which are different to those affecting males. The mortality rates are described by some as 'alarmingly high' (Malson, 1992) at 10–15%, and although some may recover symptomatically, there is concern over whether many can be described as fully recovered.

There are a number of different theories of the cause of anorexia prevalent in the academic literature. One of these, and indeed one of the oldest, is that of family pathology, whereby anorexia nervosa is seen 'in a broader context as a link in a chain of non-linear, circular, and self-regulatory interactions among all family members' (Strober, 1986). Although many emphasize potential problems with family pathology theory – that the studies are retrospective (Hsu, 1983), that few are properly controlled and that anorexia nervosa is a heterogeneous syndrome (Garfinkel and Garner, 1982) – few would deny that it has many potentially useful aspects. There are several models of the 'anorexic family'. One popular idea is that of a family characterized by a dominant mother and an inoffensive or aloof father (Crisp, 1980), although others disagree and prefer to describe a 'typical anorectic family interaction pathology' (Hsu, 1983, p. 232). Garner and Garfinkel see the family as 'culture bearers', positioning them as a 'significant force in adapting the growing child to his culture' (Garfinkel and Garner, 1982, p. 175), which, they suggest, also raises the question of whether families magnify aspects of culture and whether this might indicate a predisposition to the illness. Family dynamics and characteristics could be seen to create and maintain the condition of anorexia nervosa (Malson, 1992), but this approach alone is not sufficient to explain the complexities of such a heterogeneous disorder as anorexia nervosa. Further, lay people still endorse this theory (Furnham, 1986).

An attempt to account for the sexual inequalities of the disorder is the **socio-cultural theory** of anorexia nervosa. The fact that anorexia nervosa is more common in a particular sex, age and social class, and that the incidence of the disorder is increasing, suggests that socio-cultural factors play a large part in determining the disorder in those who are predisposed to it (Fallon and Rozin, 1985; Garfinkel and Garner, 1982). Evidence that anorexia nervosa is more common in dance and modelling students, where there is an exaggerated pressure to be slim, might support this view (Garner and Garfinkel, 1980). Many of these theorists, however, have stressed that, since many more women experience these pressures than become anorexic, the ones who do become anorexic must be in some way predisposed.

There have also been many attempts to formulate a **physiological** based theory of anorexia nervosa. One such theory considers that, before the onset of puberty, males and females are very much alike in their physical appearance and size (Crisp, Hsu, Chen and Wheeler, 1982). However, females begin developing more dramatically around two years before their male counterparts. Consequently the adolescent female, in her bigger form, attempts to minimize the difference by reducing her shape by dieting, even though her nutritional needs have increased (Furnham and Hume-Wright, 1992). Within the field of **physical** theories, particular interest has been directed towards the study of **primary hypothalamic disorder**. Hormone changes occurring at puberty have far-reaching biochemical influences which can influence eating behaviour (Strober, 1986). However, a direct relation of hypothalamic disorder to anorexia nervosa has not been established, and this approach has been criticized by many. The lack of separation of cause and effect is a fault noted by various writers (Garfinkel and Garner, 1982; Logue, 1991), who cite evidence of the recovery of normal hypothalamic function after weight gain and normal eating has resumed, the craving for food and experience of hunger that anorexics feel that sufferers of hypothalamic tumours do not (Hsu, 1983); others have criticized it for its lack of an explanation of the gender bias of the disorder (Malson, 1992).

A fourth theory which looks at the adaptation to change by the anorexic, as well as reactions of family and peers, is the theory of **'maladaptive psychosocial adjustment to the challenges of adulthood'** (Furnham and Hume-Wright, 1992). There are numerable links between food and emotion (Bruch, 1973), and meals play an important part in family life. The development of anorexia nervosa is embedded in the symbolic link between eating and emerging sexuality, biological maturity and the implications for the family (Crisp, 1980). Anorexia nervosa is preceded by a maturational crisis that the subsequent illness serves to resolve. Anorexia nervosa is seen as an attempt to eradicate the biological signals of impending adulthood and emancipation, avoiding independence and its consequences (Waller, Calam and Slade, 1989). Refusing food enables the child to stay within the safety of childhood, where others care for them as they did when they were children.

An alternative theory regarding anorexia nervosa is **feminist theory**, which has taken various forms. One of the most often cited feminist theories is that of the conflict between the traditional female role and that of the liberated woman who takes control of her own life, in a culture that praises thinness and fragility in women (Orbach, 1979). Women are encouraged to become more competitive in relation to men, and to achieve in their professional careers, yet at the same time are expected to take care over their appearance, and often cope with caring for others. Their changing bodies during adolescence are completely out of their control, and may produce feelings of confusion, fear or powerlessness. Denying feelings of hunger may be one area in which they are winning, gaining control or power. The various conflicts leave the growing woman feeling out of phase with what is going on and, paradoxically, the power to overcome hunger, to become strong, has left her in a position where she becomes weak and even more reliant on others (Thompson, 1993).

These theories of the cause of anorexia are not mutually exclusive, and several Researchers stress the importance of a multidimensional perspective (Hsu, 1983). Each theory advocates a specific therapy according to their specific constructs, but the therapies, like the theories, overlap.

Just as there are various theories of anorexia nervosa, there is a range of suggestions as to the aetiology of obesity. Some of them have points in common with the theories regarding anorexia nervosa, but the overall emphasis in the literature seems somewhat different. Obesity is described as a condition in which the energy stores of the body are excessively large (Garrow, 1986). The condition is commonly characterized by use of the Body Mass Index (BMI), a system in which body mass is expressed in terms of weight in kilograms divided by height in metres squared, and has been shown to provide the best estimates of total body fat content, correlations being 0.7 and 0.8 between the BMI measures and body fat measures of body density.

Obesity, like anorexia nervosa, is considered a growing problem, both in the US and in Great Britain, and is thought to be generally increasing in Western societies (Report of the Royal College of Physicians, 1983). The prevalence is suggested to depend on the criteria used to define it. Some have suggested that the ratio of obesity in females of low and high socio-economic status is 6 to 1, with the ratio in men being 2 to 1 (Goldblatt, Moore and Stunkard, 1973). There are many different types of obesity, some of which have clear genetic determinants, and others which may have underlying genetic factors which are influenced by environmental variables (Thompson, 1993). There are a small number of patients whose obesity is due to a specific disease or condition (Stock and Rothwell, 1982). There are also abnormalities of fat distribution, and obesity related to mental retardation and physical disability (Jung, 1991).

Twin studies have been performed in order to look at whether there is a **genetic substrate** upon which environmental influences act. Evidence does seem to exist that monozygotic twins are more likely to be of similar weights, whether raised together or apart (Thompson, 1993). This, alongside evidence of siblings from the same environment displaying marked differences in weight, has been taken to suggest that the tendency to be obese is inherited (Craddock, 1978). But such evidence does not account for the resemblance in fatness between unrelated spouses, and pets and their owners (Dietz, 1987).

There has been much interest in the mechanisms of **energy storage** in obese patients, particularly the role of brown fat or adipose tissue and metabolic rate. It has been suggested by some that obesity is a condition where the adipose tissue, the lipid store of the body, is enlarged (Bjorntorp, 1987). This is claimed to be due to genetic, endocrine and metabolic factors. Others, however, suggest that this generalization from animal experimentation may be premature (Jequier, 1987), and in any case would be inadequate to explain the aetiology or persistence of obesity (Garrow, 1986).

Several different **psychological** theories have been suggested for obesity, with some writers going so far as to say that 'in the long run, all obesity is psychological' (Dally and Gomez, 1980). Some have suggested that the obese have certain personality characteristics, one psychoanalytic description being, 'passive dependence and a wish for bigness and exaggerated growth'. This theory also emphasizes the overvaluation of food as a means of soothing anxiety and frustration.

There have also been several suggestions as to **family variables** in the development of obesity. Obesity has been found to be related to lower socio-economic class and level of parental education, and has a reciprocal relationship with family size, as it is most prevalent in only children, and decreases in prevalence as family size increases (Dietz, 1987). It has also been suggested that childhood obesity could be linked to the separation of the child from its mother (Kahn, 1973). Bruch (1973) characterizes the obese 'family frame', which is marked by much family discord and open fighting. She suggested that food can come to stand for love, satisfaction, security or power and can express rage and hate and be a substitute for sex. Such uses of food are suggested to arise from the learning that goes on in early infant-caregiver interaction (Bruch, 1973).

The **externality hypothesis**, prompted by Bruch's suggestion that obese individuals are unable to differentiate among internal arousal states and frequently interpret such states as hunger, claims that, while normal-weight individuals' eating behaviour was influenced by internal cues of hunger, obese people are affected by external cues such as the taste and sight of food. There are various suggestions as to how appetite, hunger and satiety can be affected by variables such as palatability, eating styles and situational determinants. Suggestions have been made that obesity is related to locus of control and delay of gratification (Striegel-Moore and Rodin, 1986). It has also been suggested that a number of obese patients show a distortion in **body image**, which often persists after excess weight has been lost (Stunkard and Mendelson, 1973). This often presents itself in a loathing of the body. Bruch (1973) suggests that there are previously obese individuals who may be called 'thin fat people', for whom loss of weight could pose mental health hazards.

There are clearly many different interpretations of the causes of obesity: genetic factors, disruptions in fat storage and maintenance, personality characteristics, family variables and the related learning of food behaviour, mistaken cues for eating behaviour, distorted body image, and obesity as a reaction to stress. In addition, some have suggested that lack of exercise plays a subsidiary but important part. Some of these theories seem to have parallels with theories of anorexia nervosa, as do the treatments, which are varied and tend to relate to the specific causal theory which is adopted.

This study is about lay people – in this case, a population at risk – and their theories of the causes and cures of both anorexia nervosa and obesity. Both are eating disorders that affect young people and may have serious health consequences. There has been an increasing interest during the last few years in the perceptions of the lay individual regarding various psychological issues such as delinquency (Furnham and Henderson, 1983), homosexuality (Furnham and Taylor, 1990) and phobia (Furnham, 1995). In response to the suggestion that studying the perceived efficacy of various 'cures' and 'therapies' is of practical and theoretical importance Furnham and Henley (1988), and Furnham and Hume-Wright (1992) have looked at lay theories of anorexia nervosa in the belief that this would yield 'valuable insights into the cognitive and behavioural strategies that people use when experiencing a problem or helping others' which may, in addition, 'suggest methods of enhancing the effectiveness of psychological therapies' (Furnham and Hume-Wright, 1992, p. 21). While the study of anorexia nervosa is attracting considerable interest, it might be claimed that there is still a paucity of research into lay people's understanding of eating disorders, especially the notion of obesity as an eating disorder. It would seem, then, that lay people have adequate opportunities to formulate beliefs about the causes and cures for obesity as they have with anorexia nervosa (Furnham and Hume-Wright, 1992). Some Researchers have suggested that lay and medical opinion on the cause and proper treatment of obesity varies, with lay people placing more value on the efficacy of dieting (Dwyer, Feldman and Mayer, 1973).

Clearly, lay theories are important: they are related to how people perceive those with anorexia and obesity, and the theories of sufferers could contain insights which clinicians should heed:

1. To look at the range, type and agreement with a number of statements reflecting lay theories of anorexia nervosa, and similar statements regarding obesity, in 16- to 19-year-olds.
2. To look at the factor structure underlying these responses to see which of the proposed 'scientific' theories emerge and their similarity to those found by Furnham and Hume-Wright (1992).
3. To examine the relationship between the factors found for the four parts of the study (anorexia cause and cure and obesity cause and cure) both within and between disorders.
4. To examine various demographic correlates of the lay theories of anorexia nervosa and obesity.

The rationale for this particular study is fourfold. It was hypothesized that the factor structure of the lay theories of anorexia would be very similar to that found by Furnham and Hume-Wright (1992). It was also hypothesized that the factors emerging from the factor analysis of the causes of obesity would be interpretable in terms of the major theories in the area. Finally, it was hypothesized that theories of cure and cause would be logically and statistically correlated.

Method

Participants

In total, 147 pupils attending a coeducational, state run Sixth Form College in Norfolk took part in this study, 71 of whom were male and

76 female. The age range was 16 to 19, with a mean age of 17.16 (SD = 0.60). The mean height was 68.39 inches (SD = 3.94), while the mean weight was 144.26 pounds (SD = 3.94). Altogether 46 considered themselves overweight, 17 underweight, and 84 'about right'. Nine (6.1%) said that they had at some time experienced an eating disorder, and 63 (42.9%) said that they knew, or had known, somebody who suffered from anorexia nervosa and 123 (83.7%) said that they knew, or had known, someone who was obese. Five (3.4%) believed that they knew a lot about eating disorders and 61 (41.5%) said they knew quite a lot, while 80 (54.4%) believed that they knew a little and one said that they knew nothing. However, 109 (74.1%) reported that they could distinguish between anorexia, bulimia and compulsive eating. Eighty-five (57.8%) believed that obesity was simply the reverse of anorexia nervosa. Twenty-three wrote additional comments on the back of their questionnaires, 13 of which were about the issues raised, and 10 about the questionnaire itself (structure, length, etc.). In a question asking why the participants thought that mainly females and not males become anorexic, 60 (41%) mentioned the pressure on females to be thin, 67 (46%) believed that it involved women being more concerned about their appearance than men, and 79 (54%) wrote about 'ideal' and 'perfect' images of supermodels in magazines and the media. Other ideas mentioned were those of peers and family teasing females about fatness, diet campaigns being aimed at women, sexual abuse and rape, emotional problems, vulnerability and fear at puberty and anorexia nervosa as a means of control. It was also mentioned that male role models are often more muscular and that the pressure on men was of a different kind.

Questionnaire
Participants were asked to complete a four-part, 108-item questionnaire on the subject of different eating habits. Each of the four parts contained 27 items which were to be responded to on a 7-point scale (7 = agree, 1 = disagree) with an additional option for 'don't know' responses. The first section was headed 'beliefs about anorexia nervosa – causes', the second 'anorexia nervosa cures', the third 'beliefs about obesity – causes', and the fourth 'obesity cures'. The anorexia nervosa questions were based on those used by Furnham and Hume-Wright (1992), who had previously carried out in-depth interviews to derive a list of the causes of anorexia nervosa, the

typical behaviour of anorexics, and how to 'cure' anorexics, with the most common statements being retained for use in their questionnaire. The 'cause' and 'cure' sections of this questionnaire were taken and slimmed down in order to make them more suitable for use with 16- to 18-year-olds. This was carried out in consultation with several individuals, some of whom were from the targeted age group. The chosen statements were then assessed for their appropriateness in a questionnaire regarding obesity. The statements either remained the same as they were in the anorexia nervosa questionnaire, otherwise individual words were changed (i.e. labels such as 'anorexia', 'thinness', etc., were changed to 'obesity', 'fatness', etc.), to make the statement relevant to obesity, but did not change the ideas behind the individual statements. Some of the anorexia nervosa questions had no obvious equivalent in terms of obesity and were also left out of the questionnaire. This was not common and their omission did not seem to affect the overall content of the questionnaire. The final questions were again showed to around half a dozen individuals in order to assess the questionnaire's comprehensiveness and its suitability for the chosen age group. The resulting questionnaire therefore represented a wide range of beliefs that lay people have about 'causes' and 'cures' of anorexia nervosa, with equivalent questions representing the same ideas but in a form relevant to the subject of obesity.

Procedure
All participants were asked to complete the questionnaire during the same tutorial period, which lasted 50 minutes, at their Sixth Form College. Most of the questionnaires handed out were returned, and the majority (94%) of the returned questionnaires were completed correctly.

Results

1. Factor analysis of the 'causes' of anorexia nervosa.

Table 1a shows the results of the first part of the study, the 'anorexia nervosa cause' section. The statements are arranged in descending order of agreement. It seems that there were quite a wide range of responses, and differing amounts of non-responses, from 2 to 34, which could be considered quite low. Participants tended to agree most with statements regarding societal pressures and those concerning the anorexic's beliefs that thinness is good. In contrast, statements regarding the family were most commonly rejected, and the item for which most participants replied 'don't know' (23%) was concerned with the anorexic's mother usually being quiet and passive.

These items were then treated to a varimax rotated factor analysis to reveal the underlying factor structure, following Furnham and Hume-Wright, 1992. Nine factors were found that had eigenvalues >1. Four of these factors emerged from a scree slope test as being satisfactory and accounted for 39.3% of the variance. The first factor that emerged was labelled **Rebellion**, as the statements which loaded on it at .40 and above were concerned with rebelling against parents and coping with adulthood and change. The second factor to emerge was labelled **Social Pressure** as items loading on to it were concerned with the anorexic's pursuit of thinness as a result of society's ideals. A third causal factor was labelled **Family** as statements loading highly on to it were concerned with family determinants of the disorder. The fourth factor was labelled **Coping** as items loading upon it involved ideas of how anorexia might be used to get attention in an attempt to solve other problems.

2. Factor analysis of the 'cures' of anorexia nervosa.

Table 1b shows the results of the second part of the study, the 'anorexia nervosa cure' section. The statements most frequently endorsed by participants seemed to be those concerned with psychotherapeutic treatment, i.e. those involving the development of self worth and confidence, and involving the family in treatment. Those least often endorsed were those suggesting medical interventions involving drugs and strict regimes. Treatments that were perceived to be most effective also seemed to have the most frequent endorsement. The number of non-responses ranged from 1 to 37. The item with the highest number of non-responses (25%) was concerned with the anorexic's feelings of conflict.

The varimax analysis yielded eight factors with eigenvalues>1, and from a scree test five of these, which accounted for 44% of the variance, were extracted. The first factor which emerged was labelled **Self worth** as the items that loaded upon it were concerned with promoting personal worth and confidence and helping the anorexic and the family understand her/his actions. A second factor

Table 1a. Means, standard deviations, number of 'Don't know' responses and factor loadings from the varimax analysis of Part 1 of the questionnaire: 'Causes: possible causes of anorexia nervosa and factors more likely to contribute to the development of the disorder.'

				Factors			
Statements	M	SD	Unknown	1	2	3	4
People who get anorexia think that to be thin will bring them happiness.	5.99	1.18	4		.75		
Anorexia is due to a distortion in how sufferers see their bodies.	5.82	1.49	6		.49		
People get anorexia because of a fear of getting fat.	5.48	1.43	2		.43		
Anorexia is a result of Western ideals of physical thinness.	5.15	1.70	20		.57		
Anorexia grows from a belief that to lose weight is always good.	5.04	1.52	6		.52		
Anorexics are people who are affected negatively by society's emphasis on health and fitness.	4.87	1.54	9		.64		
Anorexics are people who cannot cope with the social pressure to be slim.	4.75	1.65	6		.51		
Anorexia in women reflects a need for status and self esteem as a woman.	4.41	1.53	14		.47		
People are less likely to get anorexia if they have seen a sibling suffer from it first.	4.31	1.72	22	.42			
Anorexia could perhaps be described as a reaction to stress at puberty.	3.79	1.58	10				
You are more likely to get anorexia if food was used as a way of rewarding good behaviour or punishing bad behaviour in childhood.	3.25	1.80	31	.70			
Anorexia reflects an inability to cope with change.	3.21	1.52	15	.48			
Anorexics lose weight to get attention so that others will help them work out how to live their lives	3.13	1.66	3				.69
People get anorexia because their mothers fixed how much, what and when they should eat so they did not learn to control their eating.	3.07	1.56	17	.49		–.41	

(contd)

Table 1a. (contd)

				\multicolumn{4}{c}{Factors}
Statements	M	SD	Unknown	1	2	3	4
Anorexia reflects a desire to stay within the family and not move into more public peer relationships.	2.55	1.36	32				
Anorexia in women reflects the rejection of the role of a woman.	2.54	1.47	25	.41		.48	
Anorexics are rebelling against their parents' ideas of what is right.	2.53	1.49	8	.65			
Anorexics are trying to prove they are able to cope with the responsibilities of adulthood.	2.48	1.44	19	.58			
Anorexics come from families where the members are not very caring towards one another.	2.18	1.35	12			.63	
Anorexia results from children not being allowed to change from children into adults by their family.	2.15	1.28	17			.46	
Anorexia reflects a child's refusal to accept a mother's love by refusing her cooking.	2.03	1.38	11	.50			
The anorexic's mother is usually quiet and passive, allowing the more dominant father to control the family.	2.02	1.46	34	.60			
Anorexia results from children not being given privacy by their family.	2.01	1.10	15				.52
If someone in your family is very fat you will probably not get anorexia.	1.80	1.45	2		.53		
Anorexics cannot help becoming thin: it's in their genes.	1.59	1.10	7		.45		
Anorexics come from mainly uneducated families.	1.42	1.00	8		.60		
A person who becomes anorexic was probably quite difficult and naughty as a child.	1.38	0.75	11	.44			
Scale: Agree 7 6 5 4 3 2 1 Disagree							
Eigenvalue				4.8	2.6	1.6	1.6
Variance (%)				18	10	6	6

was labelled **Authoritarian** as it involved bed rest and drug treatments, with the doctor being in control. **Change** was the label given to the third factor, as items loading upon it were concerned with the need for the anorexic her/himself to want to change. The fourth factor which emerged was labelled **Food** as it involved the need to change the eating habits of the anorexic. The fifth factor was labelled **Freedom** as the items loading upon it suggested that the disorder itself was the concern of the sufferer and should not be interfered with.

3. Factor analysis of the 'causes' of obesity.

Table 1c shows the results of the third part of the study, the 'obesity cause' section. The statements most frequently agreed with seemed to involve many different theories, mainly those concerning food, societal pressures and stress at change. Family orientated statements were once again rejected most frequently. Interestingly, the scores were generally much lower than those for the 'anorexia nervosa cause' statements. The number of non-responses ranged from 6 to 35 and seemed, on the whole, slightly higher than those from any other part of the questionnaire. The item that elicited the highest number of 'don't know' responses (24%) was again the statement concerned with an obese person's mother being quiet and passive.

Seven factors emerged from the varimax analysis with eigenvalues >1. A scree test suggested that five of these factors were appropriate, and accounted for 50.9% of the variance. The first of these factors, which accounted for over a quarter of the variance, was labelled **Coping** as items loading upon it were concerned with the manner in which sufferers might use their excess weight as a way of dealing with various stresses. The second factor was labelled **Family** as items loading upon it were concerned with various aspects of the family of the obese person. **Apathy** was the name given to the third factor as it involved ideas of how the obese person rejects social norms and how they may have been passive and accepting. The fourth factor was entitled **Size perception** as items loading upon it were concerned with how the obese person might perceive themselves and weight. The fifth factor was labelled **Change** as items loading upon it were concerned with how the disorder might be due to poor coping abilities regarding change.

Table 1b. Means, standard deviations, number of 'Don't know' responses and factor loadings from the varimax analysis of Part 2 of the questionnaire. 'Cures: possible outcomes of anorexia nervosa and therapies that might contribute to the anorexic's improvement.'

Statements	M	SD	Unknown	Factors 1	2	3	4	5
Parents and family need to be helped to a greater understanding of the problem and need to become involved in treatment.	5.92	1.24	2	.52				
One problem in trying to cure anorexia is that the doctor wants them to put on weight but the anorexic does not want to.	5.89	1.48	3	.47				
Treatment should involve a way for the anorexic to develop personal worth and self image as being adequate and successful in solving conflict and problems.	5.88	1.23	6	.57				
The most important thing to do to help anorexics is to get to understand their way of thinking.	5.88	1.36	2	.42				
To be fully cured, anorexics would probably have to grow in confidence in their ability to solve their daily problems.	5.54	1.38	1	.64				
Anorexics must have some wish for change or escape from their illness before they can get better.	5.40	1.56	6	.44	.51			
It is important that someone who exerts some kind of authority points out that a person is anorexic as early as possible.	5.01	1.60	12	.55			.43	
If the whole family is involved in therapy it is probable that the anorexic will get better a lot quicker.	5.01	1.48	5			.61		

Table 1b. (contd)

Statements	M	SD	Unknown	Factors 1	2	3	4	5
The problem with trying to help severely ill anorexics is that they will not be able to imagine ways of getting better.	4.81	1.56	14			.54		
It is probably possible to help anorexics by telling them why they are doing what they are doing.	4.78	1.47	11	.56				
Anorexics could be said to be better when their lives no longer revolve around maintaining control over their food.	4.73	1.58	19				.61	
Only when anorexics realize they are sick will they seek treatment.	4.63	2.11	3					.62
The therapist should be clear and polarized in telling sufferers to eat sensibility to improve their health.	4.61	1.59	12	.46	.43			
A complete cure would probably involve moving out of a demanding environment into one where self satisfaction is easier to attain.	4.50	1.57	12	.55				
Pointing out a possible anorexic before you are sure could be encroaching on their right to do as they think fit with their own bodies.	4.34	1.74	22					.63
Bed rest and rewarding weight gain with greater freedom and privileges is probably the best way to treat anorexia.	4.10	1.77	25					
It is probably rather difficult to help anorexics until they are severely ill physically.	3.73	2.05	11		.41	.50		

(contd)

Table 1b. (contd)

Statements	M	SD	Unknown	Factors 1	2	3	4	5
An anorexic's mother should make all the family eat the same, thereby maintaining family solidarity.	3.59	1.70	19				.62	
An anorexic has to learn to give up demanding attention from being anorexic.	3.53	1.59	17			.58		
A good therapy would be bed rest and a high calorie diet until the patient reaches their 'appropriate' weight (calculated on the basis of height, age and build).	3.31	1.99	19		.52			
Anorexia should probably not be treated psychiatrically, as this may represent defeat and weakness and be a personal stigma.	3.18	1.73	19		.51			
The best form of therapy would probably be to take control for what anorexics eat out of their own hands.	3.14	1.70	13				.40	−.41
It is probably impossible to work on anorexics' feelings of conflict until they are at a more viable weight.	3.07	1.66	37	.41				
It is probably not necessary to have the anorexic's cooperation early in therapy; the doctor should take control.	2.75	1.73	14		.60			
The use of drugs that increase appetite is probably a good way of treating an anorexic.	2.51	1.76	15		.53			

Table 1b. (contd)

Statements	M	SD	Unknown	Factors 1	2	3	4	5
An authoritarian approach, i.e., telling sufferers they must eat, is probably the best approach in therapy.	2.34	1.71	5		.66			
The only way anorexics can actually die of the disorder is if they get so depressed they commit suicide.	1.58	1.14	8					
Scale: Agree Disagree 7 6 5 4 3 2 1	Eigenvalue Variance (%)			4.47 16.6	3.03 11.2	1.59 5.9	1.42 5.3	1.37 5.1

Table 1c. Means, standard deviations, number of 'Don't know' responses and factor loadings from the varimax analysis of Part 3 of the questionnaire: 'Causes: possible causes of obesity and factors more likely to contribute to the development of the disorder.'

Statements	M	SD	Unknown	Factors 1	2	3	4	5
You are more likely to become obese if food was used as a way of rewarding good behaviour or punishing bad behaviour in childhood.	4.02	1.71	13			.52		.43
Obesity is due to a distortion in how sufferers see their bodies.	3.75	1.93	9				.63	
Obesity could perhaps be described as a reaction to stress at puberty.	3.74	1.70	14					.68
Obesity sufferers are people who are not affected by society's emphasis on health and fitness.	3.62	1.87	9			.52		

(contd)

Table 1c. (contd)

Statements	M	SD	Unknown	Factors 1	2	3	4	5
People become obese because their mothers fixed how much, what and when they should eat so they did not learn to control their eating.	3.37	1.82	9					
Obesity reflects an inability to cope with change.	3.28	1.56	11					.65
People are less likely to become obese if they have seen a sibling suffer from it first.	3.25	1.86	15				.66	
Obesity sufferers are people who cannot cope with the social pressure to be slim.	3.01	1.98	15		.60			
Obese people cannot help being fat: it's in their genes.	2.91	1.87	7			.54		
Obesity reflects a desire to stay within the family and not move into more public peer relationships.	2.88	1.68	32	.54		.42		
People who become obese think that being fat will bring them happiness.	2.83	1.75	8				.67	
Obesity grows from a belief that to put on weight is always good.	2.77	1.63	10	.62			.40	
Obese people are demonstrating that they are unable to cope with the responsibilities of adulthood.	2.74	1.65	9		.53			.42
Obesity is a result of rejecting Western ideals of physical thinness.	2.73	1.66	21	.57				
Obesity in women reflects the rejection of the role of a woman.	2.72	1.73	14				.40	
Obesity in women reflects no wish for status or self esteem as a woman.	2.72	1.75	6			.46	.41	
Obese people gain weight to get attention so that others will help them work out how to live their lives.	2.65	1.57	11	.64				

Table 1c. (contd)

Statements	M	SD	Unknown	1	2	3	4	5
Obesity reflects a child's acceptance of a mother's love by accepting her cooking.	2.60	1.54	10			.48		
Obese people are rebelling against their parents' ideas of what is right.	2.47	1.51	9	.55				
A person who becomes obese was probably quite passive and well behaved as a child.	2.44	1.63	30			.58		
Obesity results from children being forced to change from children into adults by their family.	2.39	1.34	20	.73				
Obesity sufferers come from families where the members are not very caring towards one another.	2.39	1.58	12		.56			
People become obese because of a fear of becoming too thin.	2.31	1.74	7	.58			.51	
Obesity results from children not being given privacy by their family.	2.22	1.36	17		.68			
The obese person's mother is usually quiet and passive, allowing the more dominant father to control the family.	2.12	1.48	35	.49		.41		
If someone in your family is very thin then you will probably not become obese.	2.07	1.57	6		.63			
Obese people come from mainly well educated families.	1.88	1.43	13		.73			
Scale:	Eigenvalue			7.44	2.01	1.52	1.43	1.36
	Variance (%)			27.6	7.4	5.6	5.3	5.0

Agree   Disagree
7 6 5 4 3 2 1

4. Factor analysis of the 'cures' of obesity.
Table 1d shows the results of the 27 'obesity cure' statements. Participants seemed to prefer the psychotherapeutic-type treatments, as they did with the anorexia nervosa cures. Once again, therapies involving drug treatment and strict behavioural regimes were considered the least effective. Non-responses in this section ranged from 3 to 28; the statement with the most 'Don't know' responses (19%) was that concerning obese people demanding attention from being obese.

The varimax analysis yielded eight factors, while a scree test suggested that five factors provide a satisfactory model, accounting for 48.8% of the variance. The first factor was entitled **Understanding** as items loading upon it were concerned with the promotion of understanding in parents, therapists, and the sufferer. The second factor was labelled **Authoritarian** as items loading upon it were concerned with doctors taking control of the situation and an authoritarian approach to treatment. The third factor was labelled **Self-realization** as items loading upon it involved ideas about how the sufferers must come to terms with their illness. **Eating** was the label given to the fourth factor, as it involved the items suggesting that the obese people must control their food, and also how the problem was not a psychiatric one. The final factor was entitled **Exercise** as items loading upon it were concerned with the use of exercise in treatment.

5. Correlations between factors and various demographic variables.
In order to examine the demographic determinants of beliefs about the causes and cures of anorexia nervosa and obesity, various correlations were computed. Table 1e shows the correlations of each of the factors obtained from the varimax analysis, with each of the subject demographic variables of age, sex and size, as well as correlations with the participants' assessments of their size as overweight, underweight or about right (Estimation), whether they had suffered from an eating disorder (History), and whether they knew anyone who had suffered from anorexia nervosa or obesity, where appropriate (Acquaintance).

The variables most related to causal beliefs about anorexia nervosa were sex of participant and not having suffered from an eating disorder. Whereas females are more likely to see social pressure as a causal factor, males are more likely to consider the family as

Table 1d. Means, standard deviations, number of 'Don't know' responses and factor loadings from the varimax analysis of Part 4 of the questionnaire: 'Cures: possible outcomes of obesity and therapies that might contribute to the obese person's improvement.'

Statements	M	SD	Unknown	Factors 1	2	3	4	5
The most important thing to do to help obese people is to get to understand their way of thinking.	5.42	1.56	5	.47		.57		
Parents and family need to be helped to a greater understanding of the problem and need to become involved in treatment.	5.42	1.56	4	.68				
Treatment should involve a way for the obesity sufferer to develop personal worth and a self image as being adequate and successful in solving conflict and problems.	5.17	1.60	13	.57				
To be fully cured, obese people would probably have to grow in confidence in their ability to solve their daily problems.	5.12	1.56	8	.52		.55		
Obese people must have some wish for change or escape from their illness before they can get better.	5.05	1.80	7	.43				
If the whole family is involved in therapy it is probable that the obese person will get better a lot quicker.	4.97	1.67	3	.56				
The problem with trying to help severely ill obese people is that they will not be able to imagine ways of getting better.	4.68	1.60	11			.59		

(contd)

Table 1d. (contd)

Statements	M	SD	Unknown	Factors 1	2	3	4	5
It is probably possible to help obese people by telling them why they are doing what they are doing.	4.62	1.72	9	.59				
Only when obesity sufferers realize that they are sick will they seek treatment.	4.55	1.82	12			.69		
The therapist should be clear and polarized in telling sufferers to eat sensibly to improve their heath.	4.46	1.64	9	.59				
Pointing out a possible obese person before you are sure could be encroaching on their right to do as they think fit with their own bodies.	4.36	1.73	22			.51		.46
It is important that someone who exerts some kind of authority points out that a person is obese as soon as possible.	4.35	1.66	14	.53				
Obese people could be said to be better when they are more concerned with maintaining control over their food.	4.18	1.64	14				.43	
A complete cure would probably involve moving out of a demanding environment into one in which self-satisfaction is easier to attain.	4.17	1.68	13	.69				
A good therapy would be exercise and a low-calorie diet until the patient reaches their 'appropriate' weight (calculated on the basis of height, age and build).	4.16	1.90	7					.71

Table 1d. (contd)

Statements	M	SD	Unknown	Factors 1	2	3	4	5
Exercise and rewarding weight loss with greater freedom and privileges is probably the best way to treat obesity.	4.10	1.69	12					.57
One problem in trying to cure obesity is that the doctor wants them to lose weight but the obese person does not want to.	4.09	2.16	8		.60			
An obese person's mother should make all the family eat the same, thereby maintaining family solidarity.	3.56	1.68	17				.62	
An obese person has to learn to give up demanding attention from being obese.	3.33	1.62	28		.48			
It is probably rather difficult to intervene to help obese people until they are severely ill physically.	3.31	1.85	11		.62			
Obesity should probably not be treated psychiatrically, as this may represent defeat and weakness and be a personal stigma.	3.10	1.64	22				.63	
The best form of therapy would probably be to take control for what obese people eat out of their own hands.	2.81	1.56	15		.46			.42
It is probably impossible to work on obese people's feelings of conflict until they are at a more viable weight.	2.79	1.44	16		.54			.40
It is probably not necessary to have the obese person's cooperation early in therapy; the doctor should take control.	2.65	1.68	11		.71			

Table 1d. (contd)

Statements	M	SD	Unknown	Factors 1	2	3	4	5
The use of drugs that decrease appetite is probably a good way of treating an obesity sufferer.	2.49	1.66	11		.46			
The only way obesity sufferers can die of the illness is if they get so depressed that they commit suicide.	2.38	1.87	13		−.45			
An authoritarian approach, i.e., telling sufferers they must not eat, is probably the best approach in therapy.	2.36	1.78	4		.61			
Scale: Agree Disagree 7 6 5 4 3 2 1	Eigenvalue			5.31	3.63	1.58	1.40	1.26
	Variance (%)			19.7	13.5	5.8	5.2	4.7

an important determinant of the disorder. Not having suffered from an eating disorder was also related to a belief that the family was involved in the development of the disorder, as were larger participants. Those who considered themselves overweight are more likely to see anorexia as a way of getting attention in order to cope with problems. Demographic correlates of beliefs about the cure of anorexia nervosa showed that male participants put particular emphasis on an authoritarian-type approach, whereas older participants were more likely to favour the promotion of self worth, as did smaller participants and those who had had experience of an eating disorder. Larger participants, like the males, seemed to put more emphasis on an authoritarian approach towards the disorder.

Demographic correlates of the beliefs about the causes of obesity showed that, whereas males and larger participants regarded obesity as a problem characterized by the sufferer's passive nature, females were more likely to see it as a problem caused by poor coping abilities regarding change. Participants who saw themselves as overweight, along with those who had personal experience of an eating disorder also considered stress at times of change as an important causal factor. The variable that related most to beliefs about the cures of obesity was sex. Females were more likely to favour treatment which involved helping the sufferer and family understand the problem, and also believed that the obese people must realize they are sick and learn to come to terms with their illness, as did those who had suffered from an eating disorder. Younger participants were more likely to favour an authoritarian approach to the illness.

Table 1e. Correlations between the factors and various demographic variables.

	Sex	Age	Size	Estimation	History	Acquaintance
Correlations between Anorexia nervosa cause factors and demographic variables					
1. Rebellion	−.11	−.01	−.13	.05	−.07	−.10
2. Social pressure	−.21*	.04	−.15	−.01	−.10	.05
3. Family	.27***	−.07	.19*	−.08	.21**	.04
4. Coping	−.15	.15	−.03	.20*	−.13	−.13
Correlations between Anorexia nervosa cure factors and demographic variables					
1. Self worth	−.14	.24**	−.18*	−.04	−.19*	.01
2. Authoritarian	.30***	−.09	.17*	−.08	.11	.06
3. Change	−.08	.10	.10	.09	−.04	−.14
4. Food	.03	.03	.10	−.04	.06	−.06
5. Freedom	−.16	.03	−.07	.03	.05	−.08
Correlations between Obesity cause factors and demographic variables					
1. Coping	.14	−.07	−.13	−.03	.08	−.03
2. Family	.14	.00	.11	−.11	.12	.07
3. Apathy	.20*	−.02	.25**	.05	−.10	−.07
4. Size perception	−.06	.01	−.06	−.12	.10	.13
5. Change	−.30***	−.13	−.13	.19*	−.24**	.10
Correlations between Obesity cure factors and demographic variables					
1. Understanding	−.17*	.06	−.11	.03	−.05	.07
2. Authoritarian	.13	−.18*	.06	−.07	.00	−.03
3. Self realization	−.23**	.09	−.13	−.05	−.21*	.05
4. Eating	.14	−.03	.05	−.03	.08	.04
5. Exercise	−.03	.12	.07	−.01	.01	.09

* p <.05. ** p <.01. *** p <.001

6. Relationships between 'causes' and 'cures' of anorexia nervosa and obesity.
In order to examine the relationship between the various beliefs regarding the causes and cures of anorexia nervosa and the causes

and cures of obesity, a partial correlation was computed between all factors, partialling out those demographic variables found in Table 1e to relate to these factors, namely sex, size, self assessment of size, and history of an eating disorder. Table 1f shows the partial correlations between beliefs about the causes and cures of anorexia nervosa. The highest correlation found was between the belief that anorexia is caused by rebellion and coping with adulthood (anorexia cause factor 1) and the idea of the anorexic needing to change (anorexia cure factor 3). This causal factor was also correlated with the belief in an authoritarian approach to treatment (anorexia cure factor 2). The belief in the need to promote self worth in anorexia sufferers (anorexia cure factor 1) was correlated both with the idea of anorexia being caused by social pressure (anorexia cause factor 2) and by family determinants (anorexia cause factor 3). The notion of social pressure as a causal factor (anorexia cause factor 2) was also correlated with a belief in the need to change the anorexic's eating habits (anorexia cure factor 4). The belief that the family was in some way responsible for the disorder (anorexia cause factor 3) was also correlated both with the idea that the anorexic should change her/his eating habits (anorexia cure factor 4) and the notion of the disorder itself being the concern of the sufferer her/himself (anorexia cause factor 5) This curative factor regarding personal freedom (anorexia cause factor 5) was also found to be correlated with the causal factor which characterized anorexia as being a way in which the sufferer attempts to cope or signals problems in doing so (anorexia cause factor 4).

Table 1f. Partial correlates between cause and cure factors of anorexia nervosa, partialling out effects of sex, size, and having suffered from an eating disorder.

Anorexia cure factors	Anorexia nervosa cause factors			
	Rebellion	Social pressure	Family	Coping
1. Self worth	.14	.32***	−.23**	−.02
2. Authoritarian	.26**	.04	.10	−.10
3. Change	.35***	.15	−.03	.03
4. Food	−.06	.18*	.18*	−.07
5. Freedom	.03	.11	−.20*	.17*

* $p < .05$. ** $p < .01$. *** $p < .001$.

Table 1g shows the partial correlations between beliefs about the causes and cures of obesity. A belief in an authoritarian approach in treatment (obesity cure factor 2) correlates most highly with the idea that family characteristics are in some way responsible for the disorder (obesity cause factor 2). It also correlates significantly with the belief that obesity is a way of coping with stress (obesity cause factor 1), that it is characterized by a passive nature (obesity cause factor 3), and with the idea that obesity is a result of how sufferers might perceive themselves (obesity cause factor 4). The belief that obesity might be cured by helping sufferers and their families to understand the problem (obesity cure factor 1) was correlated with the notion of inability to cope with change (obesity cause factor 5), and the perception the sufferer might have regarding her/his size (obesity cause factor 4), and negatively correlated with the belief in the family as a causal factor (obesity cause factor 2). A belief that obesity might be a way of coping with various pressures (obesity cause factor 1) was found to correlate with the curative factors involving eating control (obesity cure factor 4) and the need for exercise (obesity cure factor 5). The belief that the obesity sufferer is characterized by a passive nature (obesity cause factor 3) is also correlated with the need to control eating (obesity cure factor 4), and the belief that obesity reflects an inability to cope with change (obesity cause factor 5) is correlated with the notion that obesity sufferers must come to terms with their illness (obesity cure factor 3).

Table 1g. Partial correlates between cause and cure of obesity, partialling out effects of sex, self assessment of size, and having suffered from an eating disorder.

	Obesity cause factors				
Obesity cure factors	Coping	Family	Apathy	Size perception	Change
1. Understanding	.06	−.23**	.00	.25**	.31***
2. Authoritarian	.31***	.44***	.28***	.33***	.11
3. Self realization	.02	−.05	−.16	.00	.24**
4. Eating	.18*	.07	.20*	.11	.06
5. Exercise	−.23**	.12	.10	.11	−.06

* $p < .05$. ** $p < .01$. *** $p < .001$.

Table 1h shows the correlations between beliefs about the causes of anorexia nervosa and the causes of obesity. The highest correlation found was between the idea of anorexia nervosa being an attempt to rebel and cope with adulthood (anorexia cause factor 1) and obesity as a way of coping (obesity cause factor 4). This belief regarding anorexia was also found to correlate significantly with obesity signifying a passive character (obesity cause factor 3) and obese people having problems in coping with change (obesity cause factor 5). A belief in anorexia as being caused by social pressure (anorexia cause factor 2) was found to correlate highly both with the notion of obese people being unable to cope with change (obesity cause factor 5) and to a slightly lesser extent with the way obese people perceive their size (obesity cause factor 4). A belief in anorexia being caused by family determinants (anorexia cause factor 3) correlated highly with both the belief that obesity was caused by various aspects of the family (obesity cause factor 2) and the passive nature of obesity sufferers (obesity cause factor 3).

Table 1h. Partial correlates between the causes of anorexia nervosa and obesity, partialling out effects of having suffered from an eating disorder, size, and self estimate of size.

	Anorexia nervosa cause factors			
Obesity cause factors	Rebellion	Social pressure	Family	Coping
1. Coping	.37***	−.01	.10	.16
2. Family	.16	−.04	.32***	−.05
3. Apathy	.17*	.13	.24**	−.12
4. Size perception	−.04	.28***	−.01	.01
5. Change	.18*	.35***	.04	−.03

*p <.05. ** p <.01. *** p <.001.

Table 1i shows the partial correlations between beliefs about the 'cures' of anorexia nervosa and obesity. The most significant correlation, indeed the most significant of all the partial correlations, was between the beliefs of an authoritarian approach to the treatment of both anorexia nervosa and obesity (anorexia cure factor 2; obesity cure factor 2). Both of these factors also had very similar items loading upon them. The authoritarian approach to anorexia was also correlated with the need for obesity sufferers to control their eating (obesity cause factor 4) and negatively correlated with a belief that the obese person must come to terms with the illness (obesity cure factor 3). A belief in the need to promote self worth in anorexia sufferers (anorexia cure 1) was correlated most highly with the promotion of understanding of the disorder in obesity sufferers and their families (obesity cure 1) and to a lesser extent with the need for exercise (obesity cure factor 5). A belief that anorexics must want to change was correlated with an authoritarian approach to obesity treatment (obesity cure factor 2) and with a belief that the obesity sufferer must come to terms with the illness (obesity cure factor 3). A belief that the anorexia is the concern of the sufferer (anorexia cure factor 5) is highly correlated with a belief that the obesity sufferer must come to terms with the illness (obesity cure factor 3).

Table 1i. Partial correlates between the cures of anorexia nervosa and obesity, partialling out effects of sex, and having suffered from an eating disorder.

	Anorexia nervosa cure factors				
Obesity cure factors	Self worth	Authoritarian	Change	Food	Freedom
1. Understanding	.42***	.08	.14	.13	.04
2. Authoritarian	.09	.49***	.23**	.08	−.11
3. Self realization	.14	−.17*	.19*	.10	.36***
4. Eating	.02	.35***	−.04	.11	.13
5. Exercise	.32***	.07	−.05	.03	−.08

* p <.05. ** p <.01. *** p <.001.

Discussion

The results of this study suggest that young people in the 16- to 19-year age group hold moderately accurate beliefs about the causes and cures of both anorexia nervosa and obesity. While similarities were found between this study and Furnham and Hume-Wright (1992) regarding the type of statements most agreed with and the consensuality of beliefs (evident from the standard deviations), there were fewer 'Don't know' responses on the whole, and the underlying factor structure of the anorexia nervosa items seemed quite different, especially in the way they related to one another.

The lay participants in this sample, like those in the study by Furnham and Hume-Wright (1992), seemed to see the factor of social pressure affecting the development of anorexia as most important. This mirrors the responses participants gave at the beginning of the questionnaire, where 41% mentioned the pressure on women to be thin, and 54% mentioned the influence of the media in explaining the preponderance of female anorexics, suggesting that this might also be the way in which many of them acquire their beliefs. In addition to the factor of social pressure, the factor analysis of the 'anorexia causes' section of the questionnaire also yielded the factors of rebellion, family and coping. The factor labelled *rebellion* has similarities with the ideas of Bruch (1973), in that there are important emotions connected with food which a person might use as a weapon against her/his parents, or which might be used by parents themselves. This factor might also be seen as having certain points in common with the theory of maladaptive psychosocial adjustment to adulthood. The factor labelled *family* seems similar to the family systems theories of Minuchin et al (1978) and to a certain extent Crisp et al (1982), and was also present in the factors found by Furnham and Hume-Wright (1992). The factor labelled *coping* has similarities with the factor labelled rebellion; however the emphasis of this factor suggests that anorexia is a result of difficulties in coping and may have parallels with the psychophysiological theory of anorexia.

The participants in this study hold various different beliefs about the possible 'cures' of anorexia. The factor labelled *self worth* was considered to be the most important and was similar to the factor identified as 'self worth' in the study by Furnham and Hume-Wright (1992). The factors identified as being concerned with food-related and authoritarian cures of anorexia suggest that young people are aware of different medical treatments for anorexia, although these factors had low mean ratings and were not supported as important, as in the Furnham and Hume-Wright (1992) study. The participants in this study were also aware of the need to promote ideas of change in the anorexic, that the anorexic must want to change in order for treatment to be effective. This suggests that young people appreciate the problems involved in trying to get people who are wilfully starving themselves to eat and gain weight. This is emphasized by the finding of a fifth factor, labelled *freedom*, which suggests that the participants in this study thought that anorexia may be seen as a personal choice and is unlikely to be treated until the sufferers themselves seek treatment.

A range of responses were also found regarding the causes of obesity, which were different in many ways to those regarding anorexia nervosa. There was a much lower endorsement of all statements involved, suggesting that they did not adequately describe what the participants felt to be the issues behind the development of obesity, or perhaps a lack of exposure to such theories. The notion of obesity being genetically caused was not widely supported by participants. The factor analysis yielded factors concerning coping, family, apathy, size perception and change. On the whole, these factors do not seem as well supported as those concerning anorexia, which underlines the observation made above. The first factor, coping, seems to contain ideas about how obesity might be a result of attempts to cope with various stresses, which might be seen as similar to ideas of compulsive or comfort eating (Craddock, 1978), notions of stress induced or 'reactive obesity' (Bruch, 1973), and also elements of personality theories. As in the anorexia section of this study, a factor was obtained which seems to suggest the importance of the family in the development of the disorder. Although this factor had certain elements in common with Bruch's (1973) idea of a 'family frame', there were several elements that were different, such as the significance of food (which did not appear to be included in this factor). The notion of the obese person as suffering from some kind of apathy was also found to be a factor characterizing the way in which young people in this study regard the disorder. This factor included ideas of how an obese person may have been passive and accepting, while rejecting social norms of the desirability of thinness, and has similarities with personality theories of obesity. A factor of size perception was also identified, which suggested that obese people somehow see weight or being fat differently, which is reminiscent of the neurotic personality theory. The belief that obesity may be caused by problems in coping with various changes in life might also be said to have similarities with ideas of obese people having certain personality characteristics. It seems that young people's theories of the causes of obesity are largely related to various different perceived personality characteristics of the obesity sufferers themselves.

As was found with anorexia, the most favoured treatment regarding obesity seemed to involve ideas of promoting self worth and understanding the disorder, which has similarities with behavioural self-control programmes (Thompson, 1993). The young people in this study were also aware of the idea that obesity might be a personal choice, which reflects the need to understand sufferers and help them develop confidence and ways of getting better. They also identified a factor that suggested that obese people would not want to lose weight and would often be severely ill before intervention was sought, which would require an authoritarian approach. Participants also supported a view that obese people should relinquish control over their eating, with doctors, not psychiatrists, taking charge of them. In addition, participants identified a factor of exercise, which was concerned with the use of rewarding weight loss and exercise in treatment. The fact that the first two factors mentioned in this section were rated more highly than the next three factors suggests that young people favour more psychotherapeutic approaches towards the disorder.

As was found in the study regarding anorexia nervosa by Furnham and Hume-Wright (1992), the most salient demographic correlate of lay beliefs about anorexia nervosa and obesity was that of sex of participant. However, unlike the aforementioned study, male participants tended to hold strong beliefs about the causes and cures of anorexia, while females tended to hold stronger beliefs about the causes and cures of obesity, although neither of these trends was particularly consistent, with females favouring social pressure as a cause of anorexia and males supporting the notion of the passive nature of obesity sufferers. Although sex did seem to be a significant demographic correlate of the causes and cures of anorexia and obesity, it did not seem to be consistently significant over the range of factors and despite the fact that males and females did seem to differ in their beliefs about the causes and cures, it might be argued that this age group were fairly homogeneous in their beliefs.

Unlike the study by Furnham and Hume-Wright (1992), significant correlations were also found with size of subject and experience of an eating disorder. Not having had experience of an eating disorder seemed to lead to a belief in the importance of family determinants of anorexia; it seems that those who have experience of an eating disorder were more likely to hold strong beliefs about the cures of anorexia and the causes and cures of obesity. Considering that most of those who indicated that they had suffered from an eating disorder will have suffered from either anorexia or bulimia, it seems that this experience has not helped them to understand the causes of the disorder, but may have helped them formulate ideas about the treatment of the disorder and may also have led them to form ideas about the causes and cures of obesity.

Neither age nor acquaintance with someone who has suffered from anorexia nervosa or obesity had a consistent significant effect on beliefs held, suggesting that beliefs did not differ significantly in the 16 to 19 age range, and that knowing someone with either disorder had not enabled the individual to achieve any greater insight into the disorder.

Correlations between the various factors yielded some interesting findings. In contrast to the findings of Furnham and Hume-Wright (1992), the anorexia cause and cure factors yielded many fewer significant correlations, suggesting that young people do not hold many beliefs that link cause and cure of the disorder. Unlike the study by Furnham and Hume-Wright (1992) there did not seem to be a belief in physiological treatments regardless of which causal factor they favoured, although between them the authoritarian and food curative factors did correlate with three out of the four causal factors. The relationship between causes and cures of anorexia seems to be more specific for this age group, compared to those in the aforementioned study.

There were also a number of significant correlations between the perceived causes and cures of obesity. On the whole the correlations seem more significant than those for anorexia. An authoritarian approach to treatment was significantly correlated with all but one of the perceived cause factors, suggesting that authoritarian approaches to obesity are considered relevant whatever their cause. However, an approach that includes the promotion of understanding was also significantly correlated with notions of obesity being caused by the perception of weight and poor coping abilities in the face of change, and negatively correlated with the notion of obesity being caused by family variables.

Correlations within cause and cure for both anorexia and obesity revealed that participants perceived the two disorders as having certain factors in common. Within-cause correlations were found between the causal factor of family regarding anorexia and both the idea of obesity being a result of family variables and of apathy regarding social norms. Clearly, the participants in this study considered the family as having an important role in the development of both the disorders. The notion of social pressure as causing anorexia was also found to correlate with differences in size perception of obesity sufferers and problems in coping with change, suggesting that social or external factors were deemed to be common to both.

In addition, a significant correlation between the anorexia causal factor of rebellion and the obesity causal factor of coping suggest that the notion of an eating disorder being used in some way, or being symbolic of something, is common to both.

Within-cure correlations seem to signify important similarities in the perception of treatment of the two disorders, suggesting that beliefs about cure are somewhat more distinct. The most significant correlation was between the authoritarian approach in treatment of both the disorders, suggesting that a similar authoritarian approach to treatment is considered appropriate for both disorders. An approach that involves the promotion of understanding and self worth also seems to be supported for both disorders, and ideas regarding the disorders as a result of free will to behave in a certain way was also a common element. However, there were important differences, especially regarding the factors of food, eating behaviour and exercise, which, although one might expect them to be correlated, were not. The similarities between these factors suggest that young people believe in, and favour, treatment which helps the sufferer (and the family) to understand her/his problem, and acknowledge the importance of the sufferer's cooperation in therapy, for both obesity and anorexia nervosa, while also believing that an authoritarian approach is applicable to both disorders.

Although the young people in this study shared some of the beliefs about causes and cure of anorexia nervosa expressed in the study by Furnham and Hume-Wright (1992), and held several beliefs comparable to the so-called 'scientific' theories of both anorexia and obesity, findings suggest that lay persons of this age group do not have a coherently structured view of the disorders, or that they hold more specific ideas about the disorders. Similarities were found between the beliefs participants had about both anorexia nervosa and obesity, with notions such as family causes and authoritarian cures being common to both. However, findings such as the decline in agreement with all of the proposed causes of obesity, as well as differences in underlying factor structure, suggest that lay persons of this age group believe that there are important differences underlying the two disorders, despite the fact that 57.8% of participants initially stated that they believed anorexia to be simply the reverse of obesity.

References

Bjorntorp P (1987). Fat Cell Distribution and Metabolism. In RJ Wurtman & JJ Wurtman (Eds) Human Obesity. New York: New York Academy of Sciences.

Brownell KD, Foreyt JP (Eds) (1986) Handbook of Eating Disorders: Physiology, Psychology, and Treatment of Obesity, Anorexia, and Bulimia. USA: Basic Books.

Bruch H (1973) Eating Disorders: Obesity, Anorexia Nervosa, and the Person Within. London: Routledge & Kegan Paul.

Craddock D (1978) Obesity and Its Management. London and New York: Churchill Livingstone.

Crisp AH (1980) Anorexia Nervosa: Let Me Be. London: Academic Press.

Crisp AH, Hsu L, Chen C, Wheeler M (1982) Reproductive hormone profiles in male anorexia nervosa before, during and after restoration of body weight to normal. International Journal of Eating Disorders 1: 9-14.

Dally P, Gomez J (1980) Obesity and Anorexia Nervosa: A Question of Shape. London and Boston: Faber and Faber.

Dietz WH (1987) Childhood Obesity. In RJ Wurtman & JJ Wurtman (Eds) Human Obesity. New York: New York Academy of Sciences.

Dwyer JT, Feldman JJ, Mayer J (1973) The Social Psychology of Dieting. In N Kiell (Ed) The Psychology of Obesity: Dynamics and Treatment. Springfield, Illinois: Thomas.

Fallon AE, Rozin P (1985) Sex Differences in the Perception of Desirable Body Shape. Journal of Abnormal Psychology 94: 102-5.

Furnham A (1986) Lay Theories. Oxford: Pergamon.

Furnham A (1995) Lay beliefs about phobia. Journal of Clinical Psychology 51: 518-25.

Furnham A, Henderson, (1983) Lay theories of delinquency. European Journal of Social Psychology 13: 107-20.

Furnham A, Henley S (1988) Lay beliefs about overcoming psychological problems. Journal of Social and Clinical Psychology 26: 423-38.

Furnham A, Hume-Wright A (1992) Lay theories of Anorexia Nervosa. Journal of Clinical Psychology 48: 20-36.

Furnham A, Taylor L (1990) Lay theories of homosexuality. British Journal of Social Psychology 29: 135-47.

Garfinkel PE, Garner DM (1982) Anorexia Nervosa: A Multidimensional Perspective. New York: Brunner/Mazel.

Garner DM, Garfinkel PE (1980) Socio-cultural Factors in Anorexia Nervosa. Psychological Medicine 10: 647-56.

Garrow JS (1986) Physiological Aspects of Obesity. In KD Brownell & JP Foreyt (Eds) Handbook of Eating Disorders: Physiology, Psychology, and Treatment of Obesity, Anorexia, and Bulimia. USA: Basic Books.

Goldblatt P, Moore M, Stunkard A (1973) Social factors in obesity. Journal of the American Medical Association 192: 1039-44.

Hsu G (1983) The aetiology of anorexia nervosa. Psychological Medicine 13: 231-8.

Jequier E (1987) Energy utilization in human obesity. In RJ Wurtman & JJ Wurtman (Eds) Human Obesity. New York: New York Academy of Sciences.

Jung RT (1991) A Colour Atlas of Obesity. London: Wolfe Medical Publications.

Kahn EJ (1973) Obesity in Children. In N Kiell (Ed) The Psychology of Obesity: Dynamics and Treatment. Springfield, Illinois: Thomas.

Logue AW (1991) The Psychology of Eating and Drinking: An Introduction. New York: WH Freeman and Company.

Malson H (1992) Anorexia Nervosa: Displacing Universalities and Replacing Gender. In P Nicholson & J Ussher (Eds) The Psychology of Women's Health and Heath Care. London: The Macmillan Press.

Minuchin S, Rosman B, Baker L (1978) Psychosomatic Families: Anorexia Nervosa in Context. Cambridge, MA: Harvard University Press.

Orbach S (1979) Fat is a Feminist Issue. London: Hamlyn.

Palmer RL (1980) Anorexia Nervosa: A Guide For Sufferers and Their Families. London: Penguin.

Report of the Royal College of Physicians (1983) Obesity. Reprinted from the Journal of the Royal College of Physicians of London, Vol. 17.

Stock M, Rothwell N (1982) Obesity and Leanness: Basic Aspects. London: John Libbey.

Striegel-Moore R, Rodin J (1986) The Influence of Psychological Variables in Obesity. In KD Brownell & JP Foreyt (Eds) Handbook of Eating Disorders: Physiology, Psychology, and Treatment of Obesity, Anorexia, and Bulimia. USA: Basic Books.

Strober M (1986) Anorexia Nervosa: History and Psychological Concepts. In KD Brownell & JP Foreyt (Eds) Handbook of Eating Disorders: Physiology, Psychology, and Treatment of Obesity, Anorexia, and Bulimia. USA: Basic Books.

Stunkard AJ, Mendelson M (1973) Obesity and the Body Image. In N Kiell (Ed) The Psychology of Obesity: Dynamics and Treatment. Springfield, Illinois: Thomas.

Thompson SBN (1993) Eating Disorders: A guide for Health Professionals. London: Chapman & Hall

Waller G, Calam R, Slade P (1989) Eating disorders and family interaction. British Journal of Clinical Psychology 28: 285-6.

Critique of anorexia paper

This research report looked at what young people thought caused anorexia and obesity, the former condition being most common in adolescence. Some would argue that it would be better to study what actually caused these eating problems rather than what young people thought about them. In response it may be said that their ideas may in part be responsible for both the cause of the problem and the response to treatment.

Introduction

Comprehensive and up-to-date, covering the major theories in the area. The study had aims rather than hypotheses; it may have been better to formulate, then test, clearly set out hypotheses based on the various theories.

Method

For both statistical and generalizability reasons it would have been desirable to have more participants: 500 rather than 150. Ideally these would be broken down by sex, age and socio-economic status as well as Body Mass Index. Some index of ethnicity may have proven useful. Overall the questionnaire items seem clear, though this study, of necessity, is possibly restricted to the more intelligent and educated young people.

Results
These were sufficiently sophisticated to explore the data but relied too heavily on correlational techniques. The authors did not relate these beliefs to the sex, age, body mass or other individual differences, which is an unfortunate omission. This was done only by correlation in Table 1e. It would have been far preferable to do multiple regressions that examine which demographic variables account for most of the variance in the various beliefs about anorexia and obesity. It is, in short, rather too much about the structure of the theories rather than demographic determinants of them.

Discussion
It is clear from the discussion that the authors see this research very much as *replicative* of previous research. There is nothing wrong with this. However, they may have more profitably considered where these theories arose from and their role in the aetiology of eating problems. They could also have speculated on cultural differences in these beliefs. However, the research does make it much easier for future researches in that a number of good attitude statements were drawn up.

Report 2

Explaining health and illness: lay perceptions on current and future health, the causes of illness, and the nature of recovery by Adrian Furnham, Department of Psychology, University College London.

Abstract
Nearly 350 British respondents completed four questionnaires derived from Stainton Rogers (1991), on perceptions concerning health and recovery from illness. They were also asked to provide a number of demographic details (sex, age, education, voting pattern) and their experience of alternative medicine. Each of the questionnaires was factor analysed to show the underlying structure. The

demographic, psychographic and individual difference belief variables were then regressed on to each factor derived from each questionnaire. Religious and political beliefs, as well as attitudes to alternative medicine, were the most consistent and powerful predictors of the health-related beliefs. These results are discussed in terms of the emerging literature on health beliefs.

Introduction

Perhaps the area where lay theories have most important consequences is that of medicine (Lau, 1982; Skelton and Croyle, 1991). Many people have theories as to the cause, and most effective cure of minor, and frequently occurring, ailments (coughs, colds, etc.) as well as major and relatively rare complaints. Based partly on their theories and attributions, lay people frequently self-medicate and give advice to family and friends depending on who is ill (Turnquist, Harvey and Anderson, 1988). These lay theories may also dictate who people turn to for advice, help and information when faced with illness, e.g. general practitioner, priest, family member or alternative medical practitioner.

According to Helman (1989), some individuals tend to act as a source of health advice more often than others. These include (1) those with long experience of a particular illness or type of treatment; (2) those with extensive experience of certain life events, such as women who have raised several children; (3) the paramedical professions (such as nurses, pharmacists, physiotherapists or doctor's receptionists) who are consulted informally about health problems; (4) doctor's wives or husbands, who share some of their spouses' experience, if not training; (5) individuals such as chiropodists, hairdressers, or even bank managers who interact frequently with the public, and sometimes act as 'lay confessors' or 'psychotherapists'; (6) the organizers of self-help groups; and (7) the members or officials of certain healing cults or churches. These advisors' credentials are mainly their own experience rather than education, social status or special expertise.

Fitzpatrick (1984) has also stressed the importance of cultural determinants of lay concepts of illness, particularly as they demonstrate the survival of forms of explanations of illness quite different from those found in Western medicine. Furthermore, individual beliefs form part of the more general system of beliefs that provides a 'coherent philosophy of misfortune'. Cultural factors influence the perception, labelling and explanation of illness. People in the West apparently seek out explanation for illnesses, such as disease, environmental factors, stress and so forth, much more than people in non-Western societies. (Herzlich, 1979)

Various analogies (metaphors, models) may be used by people in different cultures or sub-cultures to describe and 'explain' illnesses: *time running out* or degeneration, where illness is attributed to the wearing out of the body; *mechanical faults* or damage, where illness is attributed to broken or faulty body mechanisms; *imbalance* or lack of harmony, either between various parts of the body or between the individual and his or her environment; *invasion* or penetration of the body by germs or other foreign bodies causing illness (Helman, 1989).

These metaphors or analogies are the ways in which many lay people think about illness, but they often contrast dramatically with those found in Western medical science. Though these lay beliefs are complex they are frequently illogical and inconsistent. Indeed, patients may feel self-conscious about the relatively unsophisticated, foolish or even superstitious nature of their beliefs about illness when confronted by a doctor and may therefore be loath to disclose them. These beliefs are often highly idiosyncratic, being derived and adapted from a wide variety of sources. They are also highly flexible and changeable according to particular circumstances (Fitzpatrick, 1984; Skelton and Croyle, 1991). Yet these beliefs form a 'system' in the sense that they are connected to other non-illness-related beliefs and also because they are connected with the beliefs of other people in the community (Furnham, 1988).

Many lay beliefs about illness are associated with other images and ideas. For instance, Herzlich (1979) found French informants believed in the toxic influences of city life which cause physical and mental fatigue and render the dweller vulnerable to illness, while the rural environment was perceived as more natural and harmonious.

Fitzpatrick (1984) has, however, cautioned against over-emphasizing the gulf between lay and medical concepts. First, he argues that one should not forget the difference between textbook medicine and actual clinical practice, the former having complex and technical terms and the latter much simpler ideas based on selected facts. Many practising physicians retain lay assumptions and metaphors, which they use along with more scientific principles. Second, it may be that patients influence doctors as much as the other way around and that doctors use the categories, terms and prescriptions that are important to patients. Thus, they may prescribe medicines when the evidence suggests they are ineffective but which make sense in terms of the folk metaphor. Third, many patients have a reasonably correct understanding of many minor and major illnesses – their aetiology and prognosis. However, the health belief model and much of the research based on it has attracted considerable criticism (Kasl, 1974; Janz and Becker, 1984; Turk, Rudy and Salovey, 1986).

Whether guided by the health beliefs model or not, most of the research in this area has concentrated on the perceived causes of illness by lay people (Furnham, 1988). Far fewer studies have looked at the perceptions of current (and future) health or indeed the causes of recovery from illness. An exception is the work of Stainton Rogers (1991) who used a Q sort methodology to investigate what she called 'alternative accounts' of health and illness. She found eight quite distinct (though inter-related) 'theories' for health and illness.

1. The 'body as machine' account, within which illness is regarded as naturally occurring and 'real', and modern biomedicine as the only valid source of effective treatment for any kind of serious illness.
2. The 'body under siege' account, in which the individual is seen to be under threat and attack from germs and diseases, interpersonal conflicts and the 'stress' of modern life acting upon the body through the 'mind'.
3. The 'inequality of access' account, concerned about the unfair allocation of modern medicine and its lack of availability to those who need it most.
4. The 'cultural critique' of medicine account, based upon a 'dominance' sociological world view of exploitation and oppression.
5. The 'health promotion' account, which stresses the wisdom of adopting a 'healthy lifestyle' in order for good health to be achieved and maintained and illness to be prevented.
6. The 'robust individualism' account, which is concerned more with the rights of individuals to a 'satisfying life' and their freedom to choose how to live their lives, than with the aetiology of illness.
7. The 'God's power' account, within which health is a product of 'right living', spiritual wellbeing and God's care.
8. The 'willpower' account, which sees the individual as predominantly in control, and stresses the moral responsibility of individuals to use their 'will' to maintain good health.

Stainton Rogers' (1991) work is both innovative and interesting but her studies need replicating and extension for various reasons. She had only 83 subjects in her study and examined no demographic or individual difference correlates of the health beliefs and values. Apart from factor analysis, all her analyses were non-parametric and the rich data bank seemed relatively unexplored. Third and perhaps most importantly, the inter-relations between beliefs about current/future health, illness and recovery were not investigated statistically. It is precisely in the relationship between various aspects of illness/health beliefs that theories or models become explicit. This study seeks to investigate the structure of lay belief about health and illness and their major demographic and psychographic determinants.

Method

Subjects

In all, 338 British subjects took part in this study of which 29% were male and 71% female. They ranged in age from 19 to 84 years but the mean age was 37.2 years (SD 13.38 years). The average number of formal years schooling experienced by the sample was 12.2 years. In all 22% were graduates or at university. Of the total sample 36% were single, 45% married and 19% widowed or divorced. They were asked their political opinions and in all, 22% said they were Conservative, 22% Labour, 19% Democrat, 10% other and 15% not interested in politics. They came from all sorts of occupations though about a quarter were students. Asked about religion, 51% claimed to be Christian, 1% Hindu, 3% Muslim, 2% Jewish and 44% other, none or agnostic. On a 7-point scale (1 very, 7 not at all) indicating how religious they were, the mean score was 4.26 (SD 2.91)

Unfortunately no close details were obtained concerning the exact nature of the alternative medicine questioned above. In Britain Sharma (1992) suggests that five therapies – acupuncture, herbalism, homeopathy, osteopathy and chiropractic – are by far the leading alternative/complementary practices. However, the precise nature of the quality and quantity of alternative medicine experienced by this sample remains unclear. Overall this was a literate, Western sample of subjects not truly representative of the general population, being both younger and better educated.

They were also asked 9 questions (YES/NO) about related issues and the results were:

		YES	NO
1.	Have you ever visited someone who practices alternative medicine?	40	60
2.	Has somebody close to you had effective treatment from an alternative practitioner?	52	48
3.	Do you believe alternative practitioners have effective treatments?	83	17
4.	Is it only naive/gullible people who go to alternative practitioners?	7	93
5.	Do you believe there are many 'quacks' in alternative medicine?	72	18
6.	Have you ever been seriously ill?	37	63
7.	Have you ever had a life-threatening illness?	20	80
8.	Have you ever visited a psychologist?	15	85
9.	Have you ever filled out a questionnaire like this before?	28	72

Questionnaire

The Health and Illness scale used in this study was derived from Stainton Rogers (1991), who was interested in explanations of responsibility and blame in health and illness and dissatisfied with existent health locus of control studies. The 124-item questionnaire is divided into four sections:

1. Subject perceptions of their current state of health (27 items).
2. Subjects' perceived ability to achieve better health in the future (31 items).
3. Subjects' perceptions of whether they will become ill or not (31 items).
4. Subjects' perceptions of, when they are ill, the speed and likelihood of recovery (35 items).

Stainton Rogers' items were obtained from a series of in-depth interviews and from other published texts. Each item was responded to on a 7-point agree–disagree scale where 7 = strongly agree; 1 strongly disagree (they were required to circle the appropriate number). The questionnaire was also tested on 83 subjects and an interpretable factor structure emerged.

Procedure

Subjects were obtained from three sources: about 70% were obtained from two university and two polytechnic subject panels; about 20% were obtained from mature student groups and about 10% from employees from two manufacturing companies that agreed to take part. In all less 30% of the subjects were students. This was neither a random nor stratified sample and it was biased to younger, better educated people. However, it was large and varied enough to do the planned statistical analyses. Furthermore a sample of this size suggests a five-point sampling error overall. Most subjects were paid for their help and debriefed where possible. The questionnaire took up to an hour to complete.

Results
1. Perceptions of the current state of health
Table 2a shows the 27 items that make up the scale, the mean and the standard deviations. Scores between 4.50 and 5.50 were labelled agree; over 5.50 strongly agree, while those between 3.50 and 2.50 were labelled disagree and those below 2.50 strong disagree. Therefore mean scores between 3.50 and 4.50 were considered undecided.

Table 2a. Items, mean and standard deviations on the perceptions of current health scale.

(A) My current state of health is due to...	M	SD	
1. The constitution with which I was born.	4.34	1.71	
2. My body's natural defences.	5.56	0.95	S. agree
3. My state of mind.	5.40	1.30	Agree
4. My emotions.	4.98	1.45	Agree
5. 'Inner forces' of my psyche.	3.71	1.76	
6. Whether I feel 'on top' of my life, or pressured by it.	4.96	1.40	Agree
7. Everyday behaviour (e.g. getting enough sleep; eating regularly).	5.71	1.03	S. agree
8. My overall lifestyle.	5.63	1.09	S. agree
9. 'Taking good care of myself'.	5.47	1.12	Agree
10. Whether or not I'm actively taking action to be healthy (e.g. monitoring my diet, exercise, etc).	4.57	1.49	Agree
11. Good or bad luck.	2.70	1.65	Disagree
12. Simple probability.	3.03	1.65	Disagree
13. The society in which we live in Britain.	3.67	1.53	
14. The culture within which I live.	3.66	1.61	
15. The weather.	3.20	1.79	Disagree
16. My relationships with family and friends.	4.16	1.55	
17. The care of medical professionals.	3.80	1.59	
18. Whether there is somebody 'ill wishing' me or not.	1.50	1.04	S. disagree
19. God, or some other supernatural power.	2.20	1.71	S. disagree
20. Whether or not I have been exposed to infectious organisms.	5.07	1.47	Agree

(contd)

Table 2a. (contd)

(A) My current state of health is due to...	M	SD	
21. My home environment.	4.78	1.37	Agree
22. My working environment.	4.68	1.39	Agree
23. The circumstances of my home life.	4.77	1.38	Agree
24. The current circumstances at work.	4.45	1.46	
25. Particular events in my life at this time.	4.64	1.49	Agree
26. Whether or not I am being exposed at present to certain substances (e.g. pollution; additives in food).	4.30	1.57	
27. My age.			

A factor analysis (orthogonal rotation) was then performed to reveal the underlying structure of the measure. Using the eigenvalue-of-greater-than-one rule (in addition to the scree test), eight factors emerged that accounted for nearly 60% of the variance. Furthermore, the factors were quite clearly interpretable. The first factor was clearly psychological and labelled *emotional wellbeing*, while the second concerned the *work–home environment*, and the third leading a *healthy lifestyle*. The final five factors were also very clear (see Table 2b), partly because they had so few items loading upon them. Items loading on these factors were then arithmetically computed into factor scores.

Table 2b. Varimax analysis of the items that relate to the question: 'My current state of health is due to ...'.

(A) Emotional wellbeing	Eigenvalue 7.88 Variance 27.7%
4. My emotions.	.75
6. Whether I feel 'on top' of my life, or pressured by it.	.72
5. 'Inner forces' of my psyche	.68
16. My relationships with family and friends.	.68
3. My state of mind.	.63
25. Particular events in my life at this time.	.63
20. Whether or not I have been exposed to infectious organisms.	−.39

(B) Work-home interface	Eigenvalue 3.36 Variance 11.6%
22. My working environment.	.79
21. My home environment.	.76
24. The current circumstances at work.	.73
23. The circumstances of my home life.	.69
27. My age.	.35

Table 2b. (contd)

(C) Lifestyle	Eigenvalue 2.13	Variance 7.3%

8. My overall lifestyle.	.78
9. 'Taking good care of myself'.	.75
10. Whether or not I'm actively taking action to be healthy (e.g. monitoring my diet, exercise, etc.).	.67
7. Everyday behaviour (e.g. getting enough sleep; eating regularly).	.65
2. My body's natural defences.	.51

(D) Constitution	Eigenvalue 1.35	Variance 4.7%

1. The constitution with which I was born.	.84
2. My body's natural defences.	.57

(E) Societal factors	Eigenvalue 1.32	Variance 4.6%

13. The society in which we live in Britain.	.71
14. The culture within which I live.	.70
17. The care of medical professionals.	.65

(F) Fate	Eigenvalue 1.11	Variance 3.8%

12. Simple probability.	.84
11. Good or bad luck.	.83

(G) Environment	Eigenvalue 1.10	Variance 3.8%

15. The weather.	.76
26. Whether or not I am being exposed at present to certain substances (e.g. pollution; additives in food).	.61

(H) Supernatural powers	Eigenvalue 1.02	Variance 3.5%

18. Whether there is somebody 'ill wishing' me or not.	.74
19. God or some other supernatural power	.61

In order to determine the demographic and psychological determinants or predictors of these factors, various stepwise multiple regressions were computed. In all, eight factors were regressed onto each: sex, age, education, marital status, political beliefs (from left to right wing), occupational status, strength of religious beliefs, attitudes to alternative medicine (made up of the first three items shown in method section) and whether the subject had reported ever having had a life-threatening illness. These were chosen because nearly all had proved to influence health beliefs in the literature.

Table 2c. Regressional analysis of demographic and psychographic factors onto attitudinal factor scores.

	Beta	F Level	R Square
A. Emotional wellbeing			
Attitudes to alternative medicine	−.34	10.03	.18
Age	.32		
Occupational status	.22		
B. Work–home interface			
Attitudes to alternative medicine	−.30	12.38	.15
C. Lifestyle			
Attitudes to alternative medicine	−.32	12.38	.13
Age	.22		
D. Constitutions			
Attitudes to alternative medicine	−.30	10.75	.13
Age	−.21		
E. Culture			
Political beliefs	.23	7.97	.15
F. Fate	−	−	−
G. Environmental			
Age	.26	8.37	.15
Marital status	.25		
Political beliefs	.16		
H. Supernatural			
Religious beliefs	−.30	9.76	.12
Attitudes to alternative medicine	−.17		

Table 2c shows the results of the regression. On five of the seven factors, attitudes to alternative medicine were significant predictors alone, often accounting for about 10% of the variance. Because low scores indicated belief/faith in alternative medicine and the fact the beta weights were always negative, it seems that the more positive subjects were to alternative medicine, the more they endorsed the first four and the last factors. Age and class also predicted the first factor indicating that older, more working class subjects tended to endorse emotional and psychological factors as important factors in determining health. Age was a significant predictor on four factors, each time with a positive loading, indicating that older, more than younger, people believed psychological, life style, constitutional and environmental factors important. Political beliefs loaded on culture and environmental factors, indicating that the more left wing (socialist) the subjects, the more they tended to emphasize societal determinants of individuals' behaviour. Naturally, strength of religious belief was the strongest predictor of the factor labelled *supernatural forces*.

2. Perceived ability to achieved better health in the future
The 31 items making up this scale are shown in Table 2d.

Table 2d. Means and standard deviation for the second part of the questionnaire.

(B)	My capacity to become healthier in the future is due to ...	M	SD	
28.	The constitution with which I was born.	3.88	1.73	
29.	My current state of health.	4.68	1.44	Agree
30.	Marshalling my body's own strengths.	4.83	1.31	Agree
31.	Promoting a positive attitude.	5.32	1.22	Agree
32.	Actively seeking out things that make me happy.	5.02	1.47	Agree
33.	Tackling any unresolved inner conflicts.	4.80	1.50	Agree
34.	Taking charge of, and responsibility for, my own life.	5.27	1.38	Agree
35.	Changing my day-to-day behaviour.	4.59	1.56	Agree
36.	Actively changing to a more healthy lifestyle.	5.16	1.34	Agree
37.	Giving up unhealthy habits (e.g. smoking).	5.32	1.67	Agree
38.	The weather.	2.95	1.69	Disagree
39.	Good or bad luck.	2.55	1.65	Disagree
40.	Simple probability.	2.85	1.70	Disagree
41.	Improvements in my relationships with family and friends.	4.05	1.53	
42.	Getting advice from friends and family.	3.23	1.53	Disagree
43.	Getting advice from books or leaflets.	3.81	1.60	
44.	Seeking out preventive medical services. (e.g. getting blood tests, going to a 'Well Person' clinic).	4.45	1.65	
45.	Getting advice from my doctor or health visitor.	4.22	1.59	
46.	Getting advice from a practitioner of alternative medicine.	3.68	1.76	

(contd)

Table 2d. (contd)

47. Getting medical treatment.	4.04	1.72	Agree
48. My age.	3.86	1.77	
49. God's power of influence.	2.31	1.78	S. disagree
50. Any other supernatural influence.	1.62	1.14	S. disagree
51. Whether or not I am exposed to infectious organisms.	4.90	1.51	Agree
52. Improvements in my home environment.	4.147	1.55	
53. Improvements in my working environment.	4.39	1.50	
54. Improvements in my circumstances at home.	4.27	1.58	
55. Improvements in the circumstances in which I work.	4.25	1.56	
56. Particular events: what happens in the future.	5.00	1.46	Agree
57. Whether or not I'm exposed to certain substances (e.g. pollution).	4.72	1.50	Agree
58. Taking vitamins or a tonic.	4.03	1.53	

No statement achieved a strong agree score of >5.50 but the two supernatural factors did score below 2.50, indicating strong disagreement. As before, these items were treated to a varimax rotation factor analysis which accounted for over two-thirds of the variance.

Once again eight factors emerged which were clearly interpretable. The first factor, which accounted for more than a quarter of the variance, concerned *psychological reactions* while the second, which accounted for a tenth of the variance, concerned *environmental factors*. The third factor had items loading on it mostly concerned with *medical treatment*, the fourth with *self-medication* and the fifth with *lifestyle*. Once again the three fatalistic factors were clearly identified but accounted for little of the variance.

Stepwise multiple regressions were then run, regressing the same demographic and psychographic variables as before onto the arithmetically computed factor scores. Once again age (loading positively) and attitudes to alternative medicine (loading negatively) were significant predictors of many of the factors. Interestingly, there were no significant predictors of the medical treatment factor. Again political beliefs correlated with two factors (self-medication and lifestyle), and religious belief correlated with the religious factors. Again these variables could account for between 10% and 20% of the variance.

Table 2e. Varimax analysis of the items that relate to the question: 'My capacity to become healthier in the future is due to ...'

(A) Psychological factors	Eigenvalue 8.39	Variance 27.1%
31. Promoting a positive attitude.		.81
33. Tackling any unresolved inner conflicts.		.80
32. Actively seeking out things that make me happy.		.79
34. Taking charge of, and responsibility for, my own life.		.77
41. Improvements in my relationships with family and friends.		.69

(B) Environmental factors	Eigenvalue 3.12	Variance 10.1%
52. Improvements in my home environment.		.84
53. Improvements in my working environment.		.84
54. Improvements in my circumstances at home.		.83
55. Improvements in the circumstances in which I work.		.79
56. Particular events: what happens in the future.		.50

(C) Medical treatment	Eigenvalue 2.38	Variance 7.7%
45. Getting advice from my doctor or health visitor.		.91
47. Getting medical treatment.		.77
44. Seeking out preventive medical services (e.g. getting blood tests, going to a 'Well Person' clinic).		.75
43. Getting advice from books or leaflets.		.60
42. Getting advice from friends and family.		.41

(D) Self-medication	Eigenvalue 1.98	Variance 6.4%
58. Taking vitamins or a tonic.		.76
57. Whether or not I'm exposed to certain substances (e.g. pollution).		.69
46. Getting advice from a practitioner of alternative medicine.		.43

(E) Lifestyle	Eigenvalue 1.74	Variance 4.5%
37. Giving up unhealthy habits (e.g. smoking).		.78
36. Actively changing to a more healthy lifestyle.		.75
35. Changing my day to day behaviour.		.55

(F) Fate	Eigenvalue 1.40	Variance 4.1%
40. Simple probability.		.84
39. Good or bad luck.		.82
51. Whether or not I am exposed to infectious organisms.		.42

(contd)

Table 2e. (contd)'

(G) Constitution	Eigenvalue 1.27	Variance 3.7%
29. My current state of health.		.65
28. The constitution with which I was born.		.59
48. My age.		.52
38. The weather.		.42
(H) Religious factors	Eigenvalue 1.16	Variance 3.7%
50. Any other supernatural influence.		.70
49. God's power of influence.		.70

Table 2f. Regression of demographic and psychographic factors on the different beliefs.

	Beta	F Level	R Square
A. Psychological Factors			
Attitudes to Alternative Medicine	−.35	12.51	.15
Age	.18		
B. Environmental Factors			
Age	.21	7.44	.14
Years of schooling	−.18		
Attitudes to alternative medicine	−.17		
C. Medical treatment	—	—	—
D. Self-medication			
Attitudes to alternative medicine	−.39	18.66	.21
Political beliefs	.22		
E. Lifestyle			
Age	.36	14.78	.18
Political beliefs	.19		
F. Fate			
Age	−.18	4.58	.06
Attitudes to alternative medicine	.17		
G. Constitution			
Marital status	.24	7.04	.09
Attitudes to alternative medicine	−.16		
H. Religious factors			
Religious beliefs	−.38	23.94	.15

3. Perception of whether one will become ill or not

Table 2g shows the means and standard deviations of the 30 items that make up the measure. Once again, it was fatalistic factors that indicated strong disagreement and internal factors that elicited strongest agreement.

Table 2g. Means and standard deviations for the third part of the questionnaire.

(D) Whether or not I become ill is due to ...	M	SD	
59. The constitution with which I was born.	4.03	1.69	
60. If my body's own natural defences become weakened or break down.	5.54	1.22	S. agree
61. If my state of mind becomes negative.	4.70	1.50	Agree
62. Feeling unhappy.	4.44	1.49	
63. Inner conflicts in my psyche making themselves felt.	3.76	1.68	
64. Behaving in stupid ways (e.g. not getting enough sleep, working too hard).	5.30	1.20	Agree
65. Adopting a lifestyle that is unhealthy.	5.52	1.16	S. agree
66. Bad luck.	2.77	1.75	Disagree
67. Simple probability.	3.02	1.70	Disagree
68. Rows or conflicts with family or friends.	3.86	1.53	
69. Rows with people at work.	3.62	1.57	
70. Lack of proper medical care.	4.27	1.61	
71. The ill-effects of poor medical treatment.	4.16	1.61	
72. Uncaring or unsympathetic treatment by my doctor.	3.74	1.70	
73. God's will.	2.18	1.67	S. disagree
74. Other supernatural influences.	1.55	1.06	S. disagree
75. A curse or ill-wishing.	1.37	0.88	S. disagree
76. Something at home or work that I can avoid by being ill.	3.3	1.61	S. disagree
77. Whether or not I have been exposed to infectious organisms.	5.02	1.47	Agree
78. Living in a poor environment (e.g. damp or crowded housing).	4.93	1.49	Agree
79. Working in a poor environment (e.g. bad lighting or with noxious chemicals).	4.99	1.50	Agree
80. Stressful conditions at home (e.g. bad conflicts between other members of the household).	4.60	1.54	Agree
81. Stressful conditions at work (e.g. too much work, threats of redundancy).	4.69	1.53	Agree
82. Stressful, nasty or unsettling events in my life.	4.87	1.46	Agree
83. Major pleasant life changes (e.g. getting married, being promoted).	4.03	1.73	
84. Exposure to harmful chemicals (anything from pollution to other people's cigarette smoke).	5.08	1.38	Agree

(contd)

Table 2g. (contd)

85. Other people's stupid actions (e.g. visiting me with a bad cold).	4.24	1.60	
86. Inbuilt weaknesses or susceptibility to particular diseases (e.g. having a 'weak chest').	4.48	1.61	
87. The virulence of infective organisms.	5.05	1.44	
88. The weather.	3.05	1.66	Disagree
89. My age.	3.88	1.77	

Table 2h. Varimax analysis of the items that relate to the question 'Whether or not I become ill is due to ...'

(A) Stress	Eigenvalue 7.86 Variance 25.4%
62. Feeling unhappy.	.88
68. Rows or conflicts with family or friends.	.82
82. Stressful, nasty or unsettling events in my life.	.82
69. Rows with people at work.	.80
63. Inner conflicts in my psyche making themselves felt.	.78
81. Stressful conditions at work (e.g. too much work, threats of redundancy).	.78
80. Stressful conditions at home (e.g. bad conflicts between other members of the household).	.77
61. If my state of mind becomes negative.	.77
83. Major pleasant life changes (e.g. getting married, being promoted).	.52

(B) Poor treatment	Eigenvalue 4.43 Variance 14.3%
71. The ill-effects of poor medical treatment.	.84
72. Uncaring or unsympathetic treatment by my doctor.	.83
70. Lack of proper medical care.	.81
85. Other people's stupid actions (e.g. visiting me with a bad cold).	.52

(C) Exposure	Eigenvalue 2.66 Variance 8.6%
87. The virulence of infective organisms.	.82
77. Whether or not I have been exposed to infectious organisms.	.77
86. Inbuilt weaknesses or susceptibility to particular diseases (e.g. having a 'weak chest').	.56
66. Bad luck.	.47

(D Environment	Eigenvalue 1.81 Variance 5.8%
79. Working in a poor environment (e.g. bad lighting or with noxious chemicals).	.73
78. Living in a poor environment (e.g. damp or crowded housing).	.32

Table 2h. (contd)

84. Exposure to harmful chemical (anything from pollution to other people's cigarette smoke)	.56
76. Something at home or work that I can avoid by being ill.	.48

(E) Fate Eigenvalue 1.65 Variance 5.4%

67. Simple probability.	.71
66. Bad luck.	.71
89. My age.	.61
59. The constitution with which I was born.	.60
88. The weather.	.43

(F) Lifestyle Eigenvalue 1.33 Variance 4.3%

65. Adopting a lifestyle that is unhealthy.	.80
64. Behaving in stupid ways (e.g. not getting enough sleep, working too hard).	.79

(G) Supernatural forces Eigenvalue 1.20 Variance 3.9%

74. Other supernatural influences.	.89
75. A curse or ill-wishing.	.87
73. God's will.	.65

Table 2i. Regressional analysis of demographic and psychographic factors on belief variables.

	Beta	F Level	R Square
A. Stress			
Attitudes to alternative medicine	−.36	13.88	.17
Political beliefs	.16		
B. Poor treatment			
Marital status	.17	4.30	.03
C. Exposure	−	−	−
D. Environment			
Attitudes to alternative medicine.	−.29	10.12	.18
Age	.23		
Political beliefs	.16		

(contd)

Table 2i. (contd)

	Beta	F Level	R Square
E. Fate			
Religious beliefs	.18	4.39	.06
Age	−.17		
F. Lifestyle			
Attitudes to alternative medicine	−.33	16.62	.11
G. Supernatural forces			
Religion	−.34	17.98	.11

Seven factors, all clearly interpretable and accounting for as much as two-thirds of the variance, emerged. *Stress* accounted for a quarter of the variance and *poor treatment* nearly *15%*. Exposure to infections accounted for almost 10% of the variance and *environmental factors* 5%. Although *fate* and *supernatural factors* accounted for comparatively little of the variance they were quite clear. Interestingly, *lifestyle* accounted for only about 5% of the variance.

The regressional analysis showed an interesting pattern. Those who believed more in alternative medicine and tended to be more left wing, endorsed stress factors leading to illness. Married people more than unmarried believed poor treatment a cause of illness, though this only accounted for 3% of the variance. There were no significant predictors of the factor *exposure*, but three of environment. Older, more left wing believers in alternative medicine tended to stress environmental factors in illness. Religious beliefs predicted the factors fate and supernatural factors, and attitudes to alternative medicine predicted lifestyle.

4. Perceptions of the speed and likelihood of recovery
The varimax orthogonal rotation suggested seven factors which accounted for over two-thirds of variance. The first factor was labelled *medical treatment.* and accounted for nearly a quarter of the variance while the second factor was labelled *lifestyle* and accounted for nearly one-sixth of the variance. The third factor referred to *psychological issues* and the fourth *circumstances that facilitate recovery*. As in

the other analysis three clear external factors emerged, labelled *religious factors, supernatural forces* and *fate*.

Table 2j. Means and standard deviation for this part of the questionnaire.

(E) When I am ill, how quickly and effectively I recover is due to ...	M	SD	
90. Getting 'back to normal' as soon as possible.	4.57	1.48	
91. Finding ways to make myself feel happier.	4.70	1.42	
92. Finding ways to resolve any inner conflicts.	4.21	1.64	
93. Taking responsibility for myself, and doing all I can to get better.	5.52	1.236	S. agree
94. Looking after myself and taking things easy.	5.60	1.09	S. agree
95. Being careful about my day to day behaviour (e.g. getting sufficient sleep and a nourishing diet).	5.91	0.97	S. agree
96. Actively taking steps to make my lifestyle more healthy.	5.43	1.20	Agree
97. Giving up unhealthy habits (e.g. drinking too much).	5.50	1.39	S. agree
98. Good luck.	2.79	1.71	Disagree
99. Simple probability.	2.91	1.65	Disagree
100. The care I got from my family and friends.	4.61	1.36	Agree
101. The quality of medical treatment I received.	5.14	1.27	Agree
102. The sympathy and understanding of my nurse/doctor.	4.48	1.46	
103. The quality of any conventional medical treatment.	5.14	1.28	Agree
104. A curse or ill-wishing.	1.40	0.89	S. disagree
105. The intervention of a spiritual healer or healers.	2.77	1.69	Disagree
106. Prayers said for me.	2.63	1.90	Disagree
107. God's will.	2.44	1.90	S. disagree
108. Some other supernatural power.	1.61	1.23	S. disagree
109. The virulence of the disease itself.	5.30	1.35	Agree
110. An environment which is conducive to recovery (whether at home, at work or in hospital).	5.31	1.15	Agree
111. Circumstances which are conducive to recovery.	5.30	1.12	Agree
112. Particular events in my life at the time.	4.72	1.31	Agree
113. Taking drugs or medicines that are effective.	5.46	1.19	Agree
114. Treatments (e.g. surgery, radiotherapy) that are effective.	5.49	1.25	Agree
115. 'Alternative' therapies, if I sought them out.	4.43	1.70	
116. The constitution with which I was born.	4.11	1.76	
117. My body's own natural defence.	5.53	1.16	S. agree
118. Thinking positively and seeing the illness as a challenge.	5.06	1.33	Agree
119. Following 'doctors' orders' – complying properly with the treatment I am given.	5.22	1.24	Agree

(contd)

Table 2j. (contd)

120. Letting nature take its course.	4.56	1.34	Agree
121. Seeking medical advice soon enough – not waiting until the illness becomes too serious before I go to the doctor.	5.44	1.25	Agree
122. Just the chance to talk things over with the doctor without any treatment.	3.65	1.63	

Table 2k. Varimax analysis of the items that relate to the question 'When I am ill, how quickly and effectively I recover is due to ...'

(A) Medical treatment	Eigenvalue 6.39 Variance 22.8%
103. The quality of any conventional medical treatment.	.84
101. The quality of medical treatment I received.	.82
113. Taking drugs or medicines that are effective.	.82
114. Treatments (e.g. surgery, radiotherapy) that are effective.	.76
102. The sympathy and understanding of my nurse/doctor.	.72

(B) Lifestyle	Eigenvalue 4.36 Variance 15.6%
95. Being careful about my day-to-day behaviour (e.g. getting sufficient sleep and a nourishing diet).	.79
96. Actively taking steps to make my lifestyle more healthy.	.77
97. Giving up unhealthy habits (e.g. drinking too much).	.71
94. Looking after myself and taking things easy.	.64
93. Taking responsibility for myself, and doing all I can to get better.	.62
115. 'Alternative' therapies, if I sought them out.	.48

(C) Psychological factors	Eigenvalue 2.69 Variance 9.6%
91. Finding ways to make myself feel happier.	.81
112. Particular events in my life at the time.	.74
100. The care I got from my family and friends.	.70
92. Finding ways to resolve any inner conflicts.	.65
90. Getting 'back to normal' as soon as possible.	.49

(D) Recovery factors	Eigenvalue 1.82 Variance 6.5%
111. Circumstances which are conducive to recovery.	.81
110. An environment which is conducive to recovery (whether at home, at work or in hospital).	.76
117. My body's own natural defences.	.61
109. The virulence of the disease itself.	.53
116. The constitution with which I was born.	.46

Table 2k. (contd)

(E) Religious factors	Eigenvalue 1.53	Variance 5.2%
106. Prayers said for me.		.92
107. God's will.		.90
(F) Supernatural forces	Eigenvalue 1.46	Variance 5.2%
108. Some other supernatural power.		.82
104. A curse or ill-wishing.		.79
105. The intervention of a spiritual healer or healers.		.55
(G) Fate	Eigenvalue 1.10	Variance 3.9%
99. Simple probability.		.91
98. Good luck.		.90

Table 2l. Regression of demographic and psychological factors on to belief variables.

	Beta	F Level	R Square
A. Medical variables	–	–	–
B. Lifestyle			
Attitudes to alternative medicine	−.35	19.76	.12
C. Psychological factors			
Attitudes to alternative medicine	−.37	22.12	.14
D. Recovery factors			
Attitudes to alternative medicine	−.31	14.78	.09
E. Religious factors			
Religious beliefs	−.42	29.28	.17
F. Supernatural forces			
Attitudes to alternative medicine	−.27	10.38	.13
Religious beliefs	−.23		
G. Fate			
Occupational status	.18	4.79	.031

The regressional analysis showed that none of the nine demographic or psychographic variables was a significant predictor of the first factor. Attitudes to alternative medicine accounted for between 9% and 17% of the variance. Religious beliefs naturally predicted the religious and supernatural factors and occupational status predicted the final fatalistic factor.

Discussion

This paper set out to examine the structure and determinants of lay explanations for four features of health: perception of current state, ability to achieve better health, probability of becoming ill and speed and likelihood of recovery. It was assumed that these beliefs would be both related and multi-dimensional. It was, however, recognized that this 'convenience' sample had an over-representation of better educated, younger subjects, more than two-thirds of whom were female. This group was probably more likely to rate instrumental and orthodox factors as explanations for illness than an older, less well educated group.

The first striking finding was that, despite the fact that rather different items went into the four different sections of the questionnaire, there were noticeable similarities in the factor structure emerging. However they certainly did not all match Stainton Rogers' (1991) eight factors. Certain factors seem quite consistent across tables 2b, 2e, 2h and 2k. This included psychological factors concerned with either positive or negative emotional or behavioural ways of preserving or improving health; environmental or work-home interface factors; items concerning medical treatment; lifestyle behaviours, as well as various specifically external factors concerned with fate or religion. These sorts of factors have emerged from other studies using different forms of analysis (Furnham and Smith, 1988; Helman, 1989). Essentially, then, people appear to believe that the causes of health, illness and recovery are related quite specifically to factors such as: psychological temperament and wellbeing; the quality, quantity and type of (conventional) medical treatment made available; general environmental factors at work and home; lifestyle habits; societal or cultural issues; fate and religious factors. Many of these ideas can be found in popular magazines and books that seek to help people maintain good psychological and physiological health.

The fact that these very similar factors emerged from fairly different items concerned with different, but related, issues, suggests that they are fairly robust across domains of beliefs with respect to health and illness. That is, whatever sort of question one poses in this area, whether it concerns health or illness, treatment or prognosis, cause or consequence, it might be possible to interpret the various responses within this explanatory framework. Of course it could be argued that the four factor solutions were so similar in this study because of the similarity of the items and the fact that they were derived from the same Researcher. Whilst this is true, what is most interesting is the similarity between the factor solutions found in this study and those done on other data sets (Fitzpatrick, 1984), suggesting the generalizability of these ideas.

A second, perhaps equally interesting feature of this study was the regressional analysis which looked a few fairly standard demographic predictors of health-related attitudes. A number of results were noticeably consistent predictors and others not. First, some of the variables considered rarely (or never), significantly predicted health beliefs. These included sex, education and marital status. Second, strength (rather than loyalty) of religious beliefs tended to predict fatalistic or supernatural health-related beliefs, which is a sort of validity check. Political beliefs and age did predict a number of factors, usually indicating that the more left wing the person and the older they were, the more they emphasized external environmental and sociological causes and cures for illness.

Although not specifically indicated in the regression results, it is possible that as people get older they stress psychological and emotional explanations over scientific medical explanations as they observe sickness in themselves and their families. This is not to imply a 'hierarchy of correctness' with regard to explanations for illness, with the more emotional, psychological interpretations found to be associated with working-class respondents (at the one end) and the more 'scientific' explanations associated with the better educated middle class. Explanations are a function of experience, and though there may be significant differences between lay and professional groups, they are nonetheless equally valid for them.

The most consistent and powerful predictor of these beliefs were made up of three questions referring to alternative medicine: ever visited an alternative practitioner, know someone who has received effective treatment and believe that alternative practitioners offer effective treatment. In nearly every single incidence where these items were a significant predictor (itself accounting for between 5%

and 20% of the variance) it indicated that, the more subjects believed in alternative medicine, the more they believed in controllable or internal causes of health, illness and recovery (be they psychological, environmental or through a medical provider). On the other hand, positive attitudes to alternative medicine are negatively correlated with fatalistic or external health beliefs (Furnham and Bhagrath, 1993). It is possible that these results could be partly artefactual, that is inflated by method variance, because whereas most of the other demographic and psychographic factors were purely 'factual', this variable did include an attitudinal or belief variable like the questionnaire itself. However, as pointed out in the method section, not enough details about the respondents' experience of alternative medicine were obtained in the questionnaire to make a deeper interpretation possible. Yet these results do suggest very fruitful areas for future research.

The fact that a 'health' belief variable best or most powerfully predict health belief variables could of course be artefactual. However it should be pointed out that 2 of 3 items that made up this factor were behavioural rather than attitudinal. Second, religious and political beliefs seemed far less powerful predictors, except in highly specific areas. Age was a fairly frequent predictor but not as much as alternative therapy attitudes, which again is in line with previous research in the area.

Certainly, if experiences of, and attitudes towards, alternative medicine are clear predictors of general health beliefs, it suggests that measuring them is a very economical way to assess general health beliefs. However, whether these same variables predict health behaviours, as opposed to beliefs, is of course, another question!

References

Fitzpatrick R (1984) Lay concepts of illness. In R Fitzpatrick, J Hinton, S Newman, G Scambler, J Thompson (Eds) The Experience of Illness. London: Tavistock.
Furnham A (1988) Lay Theories. Oxford: Pergamon.
Furnham A, Bhagrath R (1993) A comparison of health beliefs and behaviours of clients of orthodox and complementary medicine. British Journal of Clinical Psychology 32: 237–46.
Furnham A, Smith C (1988) Choosing alternative medicine: A comparison of the belief of patients visiting a general practitioner and a homeopath. Social Science and Medicine 26: 685–9.
Helman C (1989) Culture, Health and Illness. Bristol: Wright.
Herzlich C (1979) Health and Illness. London: Academic Press.

Janz N, Becker M (1984) The health belief model: a decade later. Health Education Quarterly 11: 1–47.
Kasl S (1974) The health belief model and behaviour related to chronic illness. Health Education Monographs 2: 433–545.
Lau R (1982) Origins of health locus of control beliefs. Journal of Personality and Social Psychology 42: 322–34.
Skelton J, Croyle R (Ed) (1991) Mental representation health and illness. Hamburg: Springer-Verlag.
Sharma E (1992) Complementary Medicine Today. London: Routledge.
Stainton Rogers W (1991) Explaining Health and Illness: An Exploration of Diversity. London: Wheatsheaf.
Turk D, Rudy T, Salovey P (1986) Implicit models of illness. Journal of Behavioural Medicine 9: 453–74.
Turnquist D, Harvey J, Anderson B (1988) Attributions and adjustment to life threatening illness. British Journal of Clinical Psychology 27: 55–65.

Critique of health belief paper

There is a growing interest in health beliefs because it is argued that lay people's perception about the cause and cure of (physical) illness relates closely and logically to actual behaviours, like self-medication or consulting with doctors. This study took a questionnaire developed by one Researcher for a rather different purpose and used it to look at two things: the underlying structure in lay perceptions of health and illness, and second some of the individual difference factors that related to these perceptions.

Introduction
The introduction is rather brief and favours the psychological over the anthropological, sociological or health education literature. Much more has been written on this topic than this rather brief introduction suggests. Although the introduction explains rather briefly the aims of the research, it may have been more useful to suggest a few testable hypotheses, particularly which variables (sex, age) are thought to be the best predictors of health beliefs.

Method
As ever, the sample should have been bigger. Around 350 adults is sufficient for statistical purposes but not really for confident generalization to the population as a whole. As is often the case with studies of this kind it is the less educated, older working-class participant that tends not to be well represented. The questionnaire items seem clear and written in plain, easy-to-understand English.

Results
The analysis seemed clear and logical. First, each survey question was factor analysed, then a series of regressions were performed to attempt to determine which of eight factors best predicted the beliefs. Though their structure was clear and logical for each of the four parts of the survey, it would have enhanced the research to look at the relationships between the different parts of the questionnaire. This may have led to a more parsimonious analysis as there was clearly a good deal of overlap between the different analyses.

Discussion
The discussion section was disappointingly brief given the amount of data collected. Further it tended to be descriptive and little more than a summary. The author may have done well to speculate on those questions receiving most extra scores, or those statements where the SD indicated there was most variability in answers. The discussion could also have been more self-critical in terms of the rather limited number of individual differences measured. Finally, it is no surprise that attitudes to alternative medicine predicted best attitudes to health and illness. This is the well known problem of method invariance which forms of correlating questionnaires have with each other.

Report 3

The perceived efficacy of complementary and orthodox medicine in complementary and general practice patients by Charles Vincent, Adrian Furnham and Matthew Willsmore, Department of Psychology, University College London.

Abstract
A total of 216 patient attending either the British School of Osteopathy; a large acupuncture centre (City Health Centre); the Royal Homeopathic Hospital; or a large general practice in South London completed a questionnaire on the perceived efficacy of orthodox and complementary medicine. The questionnaire covered: (a) demographic information and experience of complementary medicine; (b) the Health Locus of Control scale (Lau and Ware; 1981); (c) attitudinal variables: belief in the importance of a scientific base to medicine, the importance of psychological factors in illness and the

possible side effects of modern medicine; (d) ratings of the perceived efficacy of acupuncture, osteopathy, homeopathy, herbalism and orthodox medicine for 16 illnesses, divided into four categories: major, minor, chronic and psychological. Whilst there was no difference between the four groups' health locus of control beliefs the acupuncturists compared to all other groups believed less in the scientific basis of orthodox medicine and more in its harmful effects. Again, acupuncture patients more than any other group tended to believe in the efficacy of that therapy to 'cure' major, minor, chronic and psychological problems. Beliefs in the efficacy of complementary therapies were associated with a belief in importance of psychological factors in illness and concerns about the harmful effects of orthodox medicine. Results are discussed in terms of the relevant literature in this field.

Introduction

Many forms of complementary (alternative) medicine have long histories. Herbs have been used medicinally for at least 5,000 years and acupuncture for at least 2,000. Homeopathy derives from the work of Samuel Hahnemann, who published his *Materia Medica* as long ago as 1811. Osteopathy also developed in the nineteenth century. Given the achievements of modern medicine one might have expected that these earlier forms of medicine would have passed into obscurity. However in the last 25 years interest in complementary medicine has increased steadily, and has been especially rapid over the last decade (Research Council for Complementary Medicine, 1986). This growth of interest has also led to more research into the efficacy of complementary medicine and people's changing attitudes towards it (Fulder and Munro, 1985; Furnham and Smith, 1988; Sharma, 1992; Wharton and Lewith, 1986).

The reasons for this increased interest and use of complementary medicine are not well understood. Some people may have become dissatisfied with orthodox medicine, rejecting its reliance on high technology, and are wary of the dangers of invasive techniques and the toxicity of many drugs. Others may retain a belief in the value and effectiveness of orthodox medicine, at least in certain areas, and yet find some aspects of complementary medicine attractive. They may regard it as especially efficacious for some conditions, as dealing more with the emotional aspects of illness, or as having a spiritual dimension that is not seen as important in orthodox medicine. In other words some patients feel 'pushed' away from orthodox medicine and others 'pulled' to each complementary medicine. Much depends on the acute vs chronic nature of each patient's medical 'career'. Further it seems most patients are quite happy to simultaneously be patients of both orthodox and complementary medicine; the popularity of complementary therapies does not appear to be solely due to discontent with the existing medical profession (Furnham and Forey, 1994). There is also growing interest in complementary medicine within the health professions. In Germany, a general practitioner is required to study complementary medicine and it is an option increasingly available to medical students in Britain; short courses are offered to practising general practitioners (Furnham and Forey, 1994). Questionnaire studies have examined the attitudes of orthodox medical students and practitioners (Anderson and Anderson, 1987; Furnham, 1993; Reilly, 1983; Wharton and Lewith, 1986) and found high rates of interest and knowledge, and referral of patients to complementary medicine. All such studies have concluded that proper and recognized training in non-orthodox therapies should be made available to doctors.

Discussions of complementary medicine in the medical literature frequently centre on questions of efficacy. There are now a number of reviews that assess the evidence for individual therapies, and review trials that compare complementary therapies with placebo or with orthodox treatments (e.g. Kleijnen, Knipschild and Ter Riet 1991; Richardson and Vincent, 1986; Ter Riet, Kleijnen and Knipschild 1990). While the methodology of many of the studies is far from satisfactory (Vincent, 1993), there is reasonably strong evidence for the efficacy of some complementary therapies for some conditions. Important though such studies are, they do not reveal anything about how effective ordinary people perceive complementary therapies to be. Research studies will gradually influence medical opinion, which in turn may influence lay opinion. However, impressions of the effectiveness of a therapy may be based on quite different criteria, such as word of mouth recommendation (Vincent and Furnham, 1993). Almost nothing is known about how effective people perceive complementary therapies to be, and yet it is probably a key factor in determining whether they will use or recommend such a therapy.

The present study aims to examine the perceived efficacy of complementary and orthodox medicine in the treatment of a number of specific illnesses and problems, of different types and severity. The present study will expand on previous work (Vincent and Furnham, 1993) in that patients attending both general practice and different complementary clinics are compared, with the aim of determining whether complementary patients perceive complementary medicine as more effective than orthodox medicine for some complaints and whether they have a bias towards the particular type they are receiving. Possible correlates of perceived efficacy and of a preference for complementary therapies, such as a belief in the importance of a scientific base to medicine, are also examined.

Method

Subjects

A total of 216 patients, 145 (67%) female, took part in the study: 46 attending the British School of Osteopathy; 47 a large acupuncture centre in South London; 73 the Royal Homeopathic Hospital and 50 a large general practice in South London. As complementary patients were expected to be of higher than average socio-economic class, income and education, a general practice in a prosperous area was selected to maximize the comparability of the groups. Initial response rate averaged 60% in the four groups, with no difference in response rates between groups. The usual reason given was shortage of time before their appointment. Mean age of subjects was 47 years (range 16–79), 50.2% were married or living together, and all groups were of predominantly (88%) European origin, and 46% were educated to degree level. Further details of demographic information by group are given below.

Questionnaire

The questionnaire was divided into three sections. In the first section subjects were asked demographic questions and details concerning their experience of complementary medicine. The second section consisted of 38 attitude statements, each rated on a 7-point scale: Lau and Ware's Health Locus of Control scale (26 questions), and four questions each concerning belief in the importance of a scientific base to orthodox medicine, and the remainder concerning the importance of psychological factors in illness and the possible harmful effects of modern medicine. The third section contained a list of 16 illnesses, divided into four categories: major, minor, chronic and psychological. Categories were derived from factor analyses of ratings of 25 different illnesses in a previous study (Vincent and Furnham, 1993): (i) Major medical conditions – appendicitis, cancer, heart attack and pneumonia; (ii) Minor conditions – common cold, hay fever, menstrual problems and migraine; (iii) Chronic conditions – arthritis, asthma, back pain and skin problems and (iv) Psychological problems – depression, drinking problems, stopping smoking and stress. Subjects were asked to indicate how effective they considered various complementary therapies (acupuncture, herbalism, homeopathy and osteopathy) and orthodox medicine to be in curing each of these illnesses, by giving a score between 1 (not at all effective) and 5 (very effective). Short definitions of each complementary treatment were given in case some subjects were not familiar with them.

Procedure
Patients were approached while waiting for treatment at one of the four study locations. The research assistant gave a short account of the nature and purpose of the study and they were invited to take part in a study of their beliefs about medicine. Complete anonymity and confidentiality were assured as no names were requested on the questionnaire. Questionnaires were returned just before their appointment, resulting in some missing data in the latter part of the questionnaire. On occasions subjects returned their questionnaire by post, but this was not encouraged.

Statistical analysis and missing data
The principal statistical methods employed were Pearson correlation, multiple regression and one-way analysis of variance with the conservative Scheffe multiple comparison test. Data were examined for outliers, normality and skew and transformations performed where appropriate.

Missing data was minimal in the first two sections of the questionnaire, but substantial in the ratings of efficacy, averaging 38.6% for each item spread evenly both across groups, therapies and illness categories. There was therefore no bias in the missing data towards any particular class of data, though there may be a bias towards a more knowledgeable group of subjects. Some subjects did not feel able to offer an opinion on individual complementary therapies, but most simply ran out of time because their appointment was due. With such large amounts of missing data, substitution of mean values or similar techniques were thought to be inappropriate. Missing data was handled by pairwise deletion of cases, resulting in a substantial drop in sample size for the analysis of efficacy data. Analyses of this section of the questionnaire are restricted to those patients who completed this section of the questionnaire satisfactorily. Subjects failing to fully complete the efficacy section on the questionnaire were compared with those who did on all demographic, health locus of control and attitudinal variables. The only consistent finding, across different efficacy variables, was that missing data was more common in younger subjects (mean age 42 versus 51 years). This suggests that the respondents are not a markedly different group from the non-respondents; it is possible that the respondents were more likely to be retired, with more time available to complete questionnaires after their appointment.

Results
(i) Demographic information and medical history
Basic demographic information on subjects in all four groups is shown in Table 3a. For simplicity, and to facilitate later analyses of covariance, data on occupation, and marital status was collapsed into three and two categories respectively. The table shows that the four groups are broadly comparable, although the acupuncture group have a (non-significantly) higher level of education and are significantly more likely to have a professional occupation. In spite of this there were no significant differences in overall income levels between groups. As a precaution, however, occupation, education and income are included as covariates in later analyses of group differences. Chronicity of illness also varied markedly between groups and, although subjects were not asked detailed questions about their particular illness or the effectiveness of their treatment, chronicity was also entered as a covariate in later analyses.

(ii) Health beliefs
Health locus of control subscales were scored and coded according to Lau and Ware's (1981) specification. People who score high on each of the four subscales believe that people can control their own health (*self control*), that doctors can control their health (*provider control*), that sickness and health are determined by luck (*chance health outcome*) and that there are many bad diseases that are not controllable by anyone (*general health threat*). The 'Science', 'Psychological factors in health' and

Table 3a. Demographic characteristics of complementary and general practice patients.

		Acup.	Homeo.	Osteo.	GP	Chi/F.
Sex	Female%	63.8	78.1	54.3	66.0	ns
	Male%	36.2	21.9	45.7	34.0	$p>0.05$
Age	Years	49.4	44.3	47.9	49.8	ns
						$p>0.2$
Education	To A level%	37.5	55.0	60.0	62.5	ns
	Degree%	62.5	45.0	40.0	37.5	$p>0.1$
Occupation	A/B%	32.6	10.3	6.5	6.0	$p<0.004$
	C1/C2%	34.9	47.1	47.8	52.0	
	Others%	32.6	42.6	45.7	42.0	Chi = 18.9
Years of illness		4.8	9.8	5.7	2.2	F = 5.55 $p<0.005$

'Harmful effects of medicine' questions had been used in a previous study (Vincent and Furnham, 1993). However, to confirm that the four questions in each group could be amalgamated, correlation matrices and a factor analysis were produced for each set of four questions. Responses for each group were highly correlated and only one factor emerged for each group. Table 3b shows the mean item scores for Locus of control and other beliefs in each of the four groups; 7 represents strong agreement, 1 represents strong disagreement.

One-way analysis of variance revealed significant differences between groups on self and provider control measures, attitudes to science and the harmful effects of medicine. Scheffe multiple comparisons revealed that the acupuncture group attached significantly less importance to science than the general practice group, and were more worried about the harmful effects of medicine than either the GP or osteopathic group. The homeopathic group, although attending an NHS hospital, were also more concerned about the harmful effects of medicine than the GP group.

As groups differed on several demographic characteristics, analysis of covariance was conducted with occupation, education, marital status and chronicity of illness as covariates. The category data for the first three variables was first recoded to form binary variables suitable to act as covariates. The results of the ANCOVA are shown in Table 3b, with only attitudes to science and the harmful effects of medicine remaining as clear differentiators of the four groups.

Table 3b. Health beliefs of complementary and general practice patients with ANCOVA

	Acup.	Homeo.	Osteo.	GP	F ratio/p ANCOVA
Self control (HLC)	5.0	4.58	4.68	4.42	$F = 1.89$ $p = 0.13$
Provider control (HLC)	4.01	4.50	4.40	4.62	$F = 2.04$ $p = 0.09$
Chance health outcome (HLC)	3.36	3.55	3.53	3.50	$F = 2.14$ $p = 0.08$
General health threat (HLC)	4.42	4.64	4.62	4.80	$F = 0.32$ $p = 0.86$
Scientific basis to medicine	3.46[a]	4.15[b]	4.20[b]	4.74[b]	$F = 6.15$ $p < 0.001$
Psychological factors in illness	6.34	6.21	6.01	5.85	$F = 0.25$ $p > 0.86$
Harmful effects of medicine	5.66[a]	5.29[b]	4.69[b]	4.45[b]	$F = 2.72$ $p < 0.05$

Means with similar superscripts are not significantly different

(iii) Perceived efficacy of complementary medicine

The mean scores (on a 1 to 5 scale) for the efficacy of major, minor, chronic and psychological conditions are shown in Table 3c; to assist comparisons between groups the overall mean scores are also shown in Table 3d. Table 3d is valuable as a summary of group differences, but should only be cautiously taken as an indication of the overall perceived efficacy of the respective therapies as a rather disparate group of diseases has been amalgamated.

Inspection of Tables 3c and 3d shows that the acupuncture group tends to perceive complementary medicine as more effective than other groups, with homeopathy patients also tending to perceive it favourably. Scheffe multiple comparisons on the mean scores from Table 3d show that the acupuncture group have significantly higher ratings than the GP group for acupuncture, homeopathy and osteopathy. For acupuncture the mean scores are significantly higher than all the other groups, indicating a degree of loyalty to their specific therapy. Homeopathic patients also have significantly higher ratings than the GP group for homeopathy, but not for ratings of other therapies. Inspection of scores for individual complaints

Table 3c. Perceived efficacy of complementary and orthodox treatments for major, minor, chronic and psychological disorders with ANCOVA

Therapy	Disease Category	Acup.	Homeo.	Osteo.	GP	F ratio/p ANCOVA
Acupuncture	Major	2.73	1.74	1.39	1.63	6.44/.001
	Minor	3.81	2.78	2.41	2.20	6.48/.001
	Chronic	3.96	3.11	2.58	2.59	6.94/.000
	Psych	3.71	2.94	2.75	2.76	3.00/.037
Herbalism	Major	2.66	2.07	2.12	1.66	.949/.422
	Minor	3.65	3.46	3.15	3.04	1.23/.305
	Chronic	3.49	3.06	2.77	2.48	2.78/.048
	Psych	3.04	3.00	2.59	2.27	.734/.53
Homeopathy	Major	2.44	2.38	2.33	1.52	1.13/.343
	Minor	3.42	3.81	3.23	2.35	1.42/.245
	Chronic	3.25	3.71	2.97	2.32	2.67/.055
	Psych	2.91	3.23	2.56	2.01	1.08/.364
Osteopathy	Major	1.26	1.19	1.48	1.32	1.40/.251
	Minor	1.63	1.55	1.69	1.39	.688/.582
	Chronic	2.67	2.51	2.73	2.36	.831/.482
	Psych	1.80	1.35	1.80	1.32	2.73/.051
Orthodox medicine	Major	3.68	4.36	3.94	3.70	2.02/.110
	Minor	2.17	2.58	2.55	2.67	3.06/.034
	Chronic	2.28	2.76	2.87	3.08	1.42/.215
	Psych	1.69	2.07	2.23	2.02	1.58/.201

5 = very effective
1 = not at all effective

Table 3d. Mean scores for perceived efficacy of complementary therapies with ANCOVA

	Acup.	Homeo.	Osteo.	GP	F ratio/p ANCOVA
Acupuncture	3.54	2.52	2.20	2.21	7.28/.000
Herbalism	3.31	2.81	2.57	2.36	1.48/.228
Homeopathy	3.07	3.16	2.68	2.05	1.46/.235
Osteopathy	1.81	1.59	1.89	1.60	1.23/.307
Orthodox medicine	2.46	2.89	2.86	2.81	.952/.421

revealed that definite discriminations were made, although the results for individual therapies are not reported here. Osteopathy and acupuncture were seen as the treatment of choice for back pain by all four groups. Similarly all four groups were clear that orthodox medicine was necessary for severe, life-threatening illnesses. Complementary medicine is seen as relatively more effective for minor and chronic conditions by the GP group, and as being generally superior to orthodox medicine for these conditions by the acupuncture and homeopathy groups.

Analysis of variance revealed significant differences between groups on 14 of the 20 comparisons in Table 3c and three of five comparisons in Table 3d. However, fewer significant differences remained after the introduction of covariates (as above). The results of ANCOVA are shown in Tables 3c and 3d. Significant differences between groups remain for acupuncture for all disease types, with the acupuncture group perceiving it as especially effective. There is also a significant tendency for complementary patients to perceive orthodox medicine as less effective for chronic conditions. However there are, once covariates are taken into account, few substantial differences *between* groups in their perception of the efficacy of complementary or orthodox medicine.

(iv) Factors associated with perceived efficacy
The fact that there are few consistent group differences suggests that there are few clear-cut differences between complementary and general practice patients. However, inspection of correlation matrices revealed that perceived efficacy was related to a number of attitudinal variables. In addition to the mean scores already discussed a mean score was calculated for all complementary therapies, and also the difference between each subject's mean ratings for orthodox and for complementary medicine, referred to as 'orthodox preference'. This measure refers to a subjects bias for or against complementary medicine, rather than their ratings of efficacy per se. A high score indicates a strong preference for orthodox medicine over complementary. Table 3e shows some of the principal relationships (Pearson correlation coefficients) between locus of control factors, attitudinal variables and mean efficacy measures. There were no significant correlations between demographic variables and efficacy ratings, in spite of their combined influence in the analysis of covariance.

Table 3e. Association of mean efficacy scores with health locus of control and attitudinal measures.

	Acup.	Herbal	Homeo.	Osteo.	Orth.	Comp. Mean	Orth-. Comp.
Self control	0.18*	0.21	0.13	0.13	−0.17*	0.23*	0.28**
Provider control	−0.26**	−0.22*	−0.16	−0.03	0.21*	−0.24*	0.29**
Chance health outcome	0.04	−0.07	−0.004	0.04	−0.14	0.04	−0.13
General health threat	−0.25**	−0.09	−0.04	0.02	0.17*	−0.09	0.19*
Attitude to science	−0.36***	−0.20*	−0.18*	0.001	0.29**	−0.27**	0.35***
Psychological factors	0.25**	0.29**	0.31***	0.07	−0.12	0.29**	−0.33
Harmful effects of medicine	0.35***	0.51***	0.48***	0.12	−0.08	0.48***	−0.36***

Pearson Correlation coefficients. 1-tailed Significance: * $p<.05$ ** $p<.01$ *** $p<.0011$

Table 3e shows that some mean efficacy scores for both orthodox and complementary medicine were correlated with the self and provider control subscales or the Health Locus of Control scale. The strongest correlations, however, were with the measures of attitudes to science, psychological factors and harmful effects. These relationships were further examined in hierarchical multiple regression analyses. Group membership was recoded to a dichotomous variable (complementary vs GP) with the acupuncture, homeopathic and osteopathic groups being joined to form a complementary group. In all analyses years of illness and group were entered first, to partial out their effects. Inspection of outliers and normality revealed that years of illness and 'psychology' were heavily skewed, and log transformations were therefore performed on these variables prior to the regression analyses.

Preliminary analyses revealed that the three attitudinal measures (science, psychology and harmful effects) were more powerful predictors than the locus of control measures. Adjusted R-squared increased very little when locus of control measures were introduced after attitudinal measures. The final analyses were therefore performed with only the attitudinal measures, with years of illness and group being entered first.

Results indicated a different pattern of predictors for each therapy. Mean scores for acupuncture as a therapy (by the entire group of subjects) were negatively predicted by 'Attitudes to science' (t = -2.24, p = 0.02) and positively by 'Psychological factors in illness' (t = 1.98, p = .05), the latter variable also predicting mean scores for homeopathy (t = 2.27, p = 0.03). The overall efficacy of complementary medicine and the efficacy of herbal medicine was predicted by attitudes to the harmful effects of medicine (t = 1.60, p = .03 ; t = 3.08, p = 0.003 respectively), while no attitudinal variables predicted the mean perceived efficacy of osteopathy. Mean scores for orthodox medicine were predicted by a positive attitude to science (t = 2.08, p = 0.02). The difference between the mean scores for orthodox and complementary medicine were most powerfully predicted by attitudes to psychological factors (t = 2.30, p = 0.02). In summary, a positive attitude to science reflects a higher perceived efficacy of orthodox medicine, whereas the converse is particularly true for acupuncture. A belief in the importance of psychological factors in illness is associated with a stronger belief in acupuncture and homeopathy, and is the crucial distinguishing factor in predicting efficacy of complementary medicine in relation to beliefs in orthodox medicine.

Discussion
Previous comparisons of locus of control in complementary and general practice groups have found that where differences arose certain patients of complementary medicine, namely homeopathy, tend to have less significant beliefs about provider control; that is that doctors cure illness (Furnham and Smith, 1988) and more significant beliefs about self control; that is that they themselves are the major cause of both health and illness (Furnham and Bhagrath, 1993). It is only these two scales which in the past have revealed significant differences. Similarly, in this study we found differences only on the self and provider control subscales, but these did not remain significant after the introduction of demographic covariates. Only attitudes to science and beliefs in the harmful effects of medicine clearly differentiated the four groups after analysis of covariance. This suggests that these attitudinal variables may be more important characteristics to study, when attempting to understand complementary medicine, than the locus of control beliefs examined in previous studies. Differences between groups even on these variables,

however, are relatively small. There is no evidence of a 'flight from science' characterizing all complementary patients.

Orthodox medicine was seen by all patients, whether GP or complementary, as being more effective in the treatment of major, life-threatening, conditions. This was in agreement with previous work in this field (Furnham, 1992; Furnham and Forey, 1994). Complementary medicine was seen as more effective in the treatment of chronic and minor conditions by the acupuncture and homeopathy groups, and relatively more effective by the GP group. For some conditions some form of complementary medicine was seen as the most effective treatment by all patients. Osteopathy and acupuncture are both seen as especially useful in the treatment of back pain, and herbalism is seen as a valid treatment for fatigue and stress, or at least orthodox treatment is seen as particularly ineffective for these complaints.

Many of the more complex ratings of efficacy were incomplete (shortage of time again) and this data must be treated with considerable caution, until follow-up studies have been carried out. However, only age differentiated responders and non-responders to the efficacy ratings; there was no evidence of any important bias in this respect.

Perceptions of efficacy were also compared across the four groups, with many significant differences initially found. However, the introduction of covariates (occupation, education, marital status and chronicity of illness) to control for group differences reduced the number of significant comparisons. However, complementary medicine still tended to be perceived as relatively more effective for chronic conditions by the complementary group, and pronounced group differences were seen in perceptions of acupuncture. This latter result seems to indicate a particular loyalty to their therapy on the part of these acupuncture patients. This may reflect a different referral pattern (more self-selection, less referral) or a different attitude to complementary medicine in this especially traditionally oriented centre.

The study and analysis of group differences, between complementary and GP patients, is a ideally a prelude and a means to understanding the factors that underlie perceived efficacy. The fact that there were relatively few consistent group difference suggested that there are few clear cut differences between complementary and general practice patients. There is, in other words, no stereotypic 'complementary patient'. We therefore examined other possible correlates of perceived efficacy. Regression analyses indicated that locus of control measures were at best a secondary factor. The importance of a scientific base to medicine, the importance of psychological factors in illness and the potential harmful effects of medicine all appeared as predictors in regression analyses, although their relative importance varied according to the therapy under discussion. Positive attitudes to science were associated with stronger beliefs in orthodox medicine and weaker beliefs in acupuncture. A belief in the harmful effects of orthodox medicine was associated with a greater belief in the efficacy of herbal medicine. The most powerful overall predictor, clearly associated with a relative preference for complementary medicine, related to a belief in the importance of psychological factors in illness. This suggests, not that complementary therapies are viewed as placebos, but that patients may be drawn to complementary medicine because it is seen as more able to take a psychological perspective into account. Some complementary therapies (e.g. homeopathy, some forms of acupuncture) explicitly take emotional factors into account in their diagnoses and underlying theory, though it is not clear how far this matters (or is indeed noticed by) most patients. It may be complementary practitioners simply have more time, or are seen to be more receptive to discussing emotional aspects of illness.

We have already acknowledged that the perceived efficacy data is flawed and incomplete. The results are nevertheless of interest, and the method of enquiry is valuable. Future studies should use a simplified and shorter assessment of relative efficacy, less ambitious in the number of comparisons attempted and the range of therapies surveyed. We also suggest that straightforward group comparisons are not the optimal method of enquiry, although different groups should be surveyed. Future studies should concentrate on relating perceived efficacy to more basic attitudinal variables, though with the proviso that the relationships may vary in different patient groups.

Acknowledgments

We are grateful to the Research Council for Complementary Medicine for supporting the study. We thank the following people for assisting with the study: Dr Todd and the reception staff at Raynes Park Surgery; Dr Fisher at the Royal National Homeopathic

Hospital; Research staff and receptionists at the British School of Osteopathy; Geoff Wadlow and staff at the City Health Centre.

References

Anderson E, Anderson, P (1987) General practitioners and alternative medicine. Journal of Royal College of General Practitioners 37: 52–5.

Fulder S, Munro R (1985) Complementary medicine in the United Kingdom: Patients, practitioners and consultants. Lancet 8454: 542–5.

Furnham A (1993) Attitudes to alternative medicine: a study of the perception of those studying orthodox medicine. Complementary Therapies in Medicine 1: 120–6.

Furnham A, Bhagrath R (1993) A comparison of health beliefs and behaviours of clients of orthodox and complementary medicine. British Journal of Clinical Psychology 32: 237–46.

Furnham A, Forey J (1994) The attitudes, behaviours and beliefs of patients of conventional vs complementary (alternative) medicine. Journal of Clinical Psychology 50:.458–69.

Furnham A, Smith C (1988) Choosing alternative medicine: A comparison of the beliefs of patients visiting a GP and a homeopath. Social Science and Medicine 26: 685–7.

Kleijnen J, Knipschild P, Ter Riet G (1991) Clinical trials of homeopathy. British Medical Journal 302: 316–23.

Lau R, Ware K (1981) Refinements in the measurement of health-specific locus-of-control beliefs. Medical Care 19: 1147–58.

Richardson PH, Vincent CA (1986) Acupuncture for the treatment of chronic pain: a review of evaluative research. Pain 24: 15–40.

Reilly D (1983) 'Young doctors' views on alternative medicine. British Medical Journal 287: 337–9.

Sharma U (1992) Complementary Medicine Today: Practitioners and Patients. London: Routledge.

Ter Riet G, Kleijnen J, Knipschild P (1990) Acupuncture and chronic pain: a criterion based meta-analysis. Journal of Clinical Epidemiology 11: 1191–9.

Vincent CA (1993) Acupuncture. In Lewith GT, Aldridge DA (eds) Clinical Research Methodology. London, Hodder and Stoughton.

Vincent CA, Furnham A (1993) The perceived efficacy of orthodox and complementary medicine. Unpublished paper.

Wharton R, Lewith G (1986) Complementary medicine and the general practitioner. British Medical Journal 992: 1498–500.

Critique of complementary medicine paper

This research paper reported on a modest replication of an equally modest earlier paper in the neglected but fast-growing area of complementary medicine. It examined how different complementary medicine patients assessed the efficacy of their preferred treatment, together with other major specialisms in curing specific illnesses. It also looked at the relationship between attitudes to medicine and the perception of efficacy of methods.

Introduction
This was brief and to the point, but the paper only quotes 12 references in all! A more comprehensive and critical introduction may well have reviewed two to three times as many papers salient to this topic. The research has, however, a very simple aim: to see if a previous very similar study could be replicated in a different and bigger population with better compliance figures.

Method
The major problem with this study is the very limited number of participants – only 82. At least 400 should have taken part. Further, it would have been preferable to gather details on the participants' traditional demographic factors (age, sex, occupation), history of illness, as well as exposure to alternative medicine practitioners. Although some of these facts were gathered, they were not systematically included in the analysis.

Results
This was very clear, though it is not spelt out how the 12 illnesses specified were categorized into the few groups: chronic, major, minor and psychological.

Discussion
Clear and descriptive but not linked to the results from other relevant studies in this area. The paper may also have usefully been more self-critical.

References

The book by A. Oppenheim is the most readable and often considered to be the best of the major books on survey, questionnaire and interview techniques. It is therefore the recommended further text for those seriously interested in survey design. Readers should refer to the references provided in the three example reports for that background material.

Anastasi A (1988) Psychological Testing. USA: Macmillan.
Babbie ER (1973) Survey Research Methods. USA: Wadsworth Publishing Co.
Bowling A (1995) Measuring Disease. UK: Open University Press
Cook JD, Hepworth SJ, Wall TD, Warr P (1981) The Experience of Work: A Compendium and Review of 249 Measures and Their Use. London: Academic Press.
Couchman W, Dawson J (1990) Nursing and Health-care Research. UK: Scutari Press.
De Vaus DA (1991) Surveys in Social Research. UK: UCL Press.
Edwards JE, Thomas MD, Rosenfeld P, Booth-Kewley, S (1997) How to Conduct Organizational Surveys: A Step by Step Guide. USA: Sage.
Fink A, Cosec J (1985) How to Conduct Surveys. USA: Sage.
Foddy W (1995) Constructing Questions for Interviews and Questionnaires. USA: Cambridge University Press.
Furnham A (1994) The Barnum effect in medicine. Complementary Therapies in Medicine 2: 1–4.
Furnham A (1995) Lay beliefs about phobia. Journal of Clinical Psychology 51: 518–25.
Furnham A, Bower P (1992) A comparison of academic and lay theories of schizophrenia. British Journal of Psychiatry 161: 201–10.
Furnham A, Thompson L (1996) Lay theories of heroin addiction. Soc Sci Med 43: 29–40.
Gaugler BB, Rosenthal DB, Thornton GC, Bentson C (1987) Meta Analysis of Assessment Centre Validity 72: 493–511.
Henry G (1990) Practical Sampling. Newbury Park, CA: Sage.
Kline P (1986) Handbook of Test Construction. UK: Methuen.

References

Kline P (1993) The handbook of psychological testing. UK: Routledge.

Kline P (1994) An Easy Guide to Factor Analysis. London: Routledge.

Lavrakas PJ (1987) Telephone Survey Methods. USA: Sage.

Marks D, Kammann R (1980) The Psychology of the Psychic. Buffalo, NY: Prometheus Books.

McDowell I, Newell C (1987) Measuring Health: A Guide to Rating Scales and Questionnaires. UK: Oxford University Press.

Moser CA, Kalton G (1971) Survey Methods in Social Investigation. UK: Heinemann Educational.

Nachmias C, Nachmias D (1981) Research Methods in the Social Sciences. UK: Edward Arnold Publishers Ltd.

Oppenheim A (1992) Questionnaire Design, Interviewing and Attitude Measurement. UK: Pinters Publishers.

Pearson A (Ed) (1988) Nursing Quality Measurement. UK: John Wiley & Sons.

Polit DF, Hungler B (1991) Nursing Research: Principles and Methods. USA: JB Lippincott Co.

Rea L, Parker R (1992) Designing and Conducting Survey Research: A Comprehensive Guide. San Francisco: Jossey-Bass.

Rosenberg M (1968) The Logic of Survey Analysis. USA: Basic Books.

Rust J, Golombok S (1989) Modern Psychometrics. UK: Routledge.

Sapsford R, Abbott P (1992) Research Methods for Nurses and the Caring Professions. UK: Open University.

Schuman H, Presser S (1981) Questions and Answers in Attitude Surveys. USA: Academic Press.

Wellings K, Field J, Johnson A, Wadsworth J, Bradshaw S (1994) Sexual Behaviour in Britain. UK: Penguin.

Wiles A Quality of patient care scale. In Pearson A (1988) Nursing Quality Measurement. UK: John Wiley and Sons.

Wilson P, Spence S, Kavangh D (1989) Cognitive Behavioural Interviewing for Adult Disorders. London: Routledge.

Index

abstract, in report 185–186, 192
abstract qualities, measuring 13
abstracts, using for research 59
acceptability of items and format 100, 116–117
acting on survey results 5, 10, 15, 29–30
additive scales 123–124
adjectives, rank scale 123
administration method, surveys 9, 89–91
American Psychological Association, code of conduct 27
analysis *see* data, analysis
anonymity, respondents 15, 74, 78, 90, 113–114
anorexia report 198–234
  critique 234–235
ANOVA 156, 173
  repeated measures 156, 173
astrology 142–143, 194–195
attribution errors 146
audiovisual techniques 189
authorization, obtaining 50, 95
averages 156, 157, 161–163

bar graphs 187–188
Barnum effect 143
'before and after' studies 66
bell-shaped curve 160
beneficence 27
best practice 10–11, 50, 103, 132, 172, 185

bias
  and causality 66
  and consent 30
  eliminating 129–130
  interviewer 90
  personal 112, 146
  potential 189
  and wording of questionnaire 116–117
biased sample, definition 92
blind evaluation 4
brainstorming 104
British Psychological Society, code of conduct 27

cancer patients, quality of life questionnaires 35–36
cardiovascular diseases, quality of life measurements 41–42
catchphrases 118–120
categories, clear 12
category scale 121–122, 156
causality 66–67, 171, 189–190
central tendency *see* average
change
  before and after studies 66
  in organization 7
cheating or faking 129–131, 145, 148, 189
checking, researcher's responsibility 132
checklist 120–121
chi-square 156, 172

clarity
    of objectives 12
    of survey item formulation
        124–125
    of wording 21
client
    commitment 8
    definition xii
    needs 13
    objective 20–22
clinical trials 70
closed questions 116–120
codes of conduct 27
coding, and data entry 131–132
cohort designs 69
colloquialisms, avoiding 124–125
comparisons 172–173
complementary and orthodox medicine report 260–274
    critique 274–275
computer methods
    factor rotation 179
    presentation software 189
    spreadsheets 131, 180–181
    statistical analysis 9, 91, 153, 154, 172, 180–181
    survey administration 82–83, 90–91
    telephone interviews 89
concurrent validity 147, 148
confidence intervals 172
confidentiality, respondents 15, 48, 74, 78
consent, respondents 28, 30
consistency 146
construct validity 147–148, 149
content analysis 115
content areas 105, 112
content validity 147, 148
contingency tables 167, 168
continuous data 156, 164, 166
contrasting people 101
control group 4, 65–66, 70
correlation
    and causation 171
    coefficient 168, 169, 171, 173
    and factor loading 175
    negative and positive 169–171

costs
    computerised survey methods 90–91
    focus groups 102
    interview method 87, 89
    planning 8
    surveys 3, 14, 44, 49
    telephone surveys 84
covering letter, in postal survey 73, 75–76, 77
covert methods 28, 33
creativity 100
credibility of sampling 79, 93
criterion
    appropriateness 144
    identifying 143–144
    test 147
criticism, responding to 13–15, 189–190
critiques
    anorexia and obesity report 234–235
    complementary and orthodox medicine report 274–275
    lay perceptions of health and illness report 259–260
Cronbach's alpha 140–141, 180
cross-sectional survey design 66–68, 156
cross-tabulations 157
culture
    occupational groups 61
    organisation 6–7
cumulative frequency distribution 160–161
current practice, determining 61
cutting corners 10, 44, 50

data
    analysis
        computerised 9, 180–181
        expert help 54, 154
        methods 156
        planning 153
    in decision-making 3
    entry
        by respondent 82, 132
        and coding 131–132
        cost 49

Index

incomplete 83, 125
objective 33
obtaining without a survey 31–33
quantifiable 4
unbiased 4–5, 84
deception *see* cheating and faking;
    covert methods
decision-making, data 3
definition of terms xi–xii, 92
dependent and independent variables
    173
descriptive statistics 59–60, 157–166
design
    cohort 69
    cross-sectional 66–68
    experimental 65–66, 69–71
    longitudinal 68–69
    non-experimental descriptive 65,
        66–69
    normative 66
    panel 69
    quasi-experimental 65–66, 69–71
    trend 68
design, *see also* questionnaire, format
dimensions *see* categories
direct interviews 83
disclosure 28
disease-related quality of life
    measurements 43
disks, for computer administered
    surveys 83
distribution
    asymmetrical 160
    curve 139–140, 159–160
    modality 160
    symmetrical 159–160
'don't know' answers 120, 125
double negatives, avoiding 116

eigenvalues greater than 1 110, 179
embarrassment of respondents 125
equal probability sampling 93–94
equipment and buildings, assessing 6
errors
    simple random sampling 93–94
    sums of squares 174
ethical considerations
    clinical trials 70
    planning 8

sponsorship 76
surveys 27–32, 74, 195–196
ethics committee 28–29
evaluation
    blind 4
    consent to 30
    objective and subjective 3
    of organisations 5
example reports 198–275
Excel *see* spreadsheets
experimental design 65–66, 69–71
expert group 138, 148
expert help, data analysis 54, 154
expert help, *see also* subject experts
exploratory factor analysis 109–110

face validity 141–143, 148
fact-based survey, qualitative trial run
    137–138, 149
factor
    analysis 175–180
        exploratory 109–110
    how many to use 177, 179
    loading 175, 177–178
    rotation 110, 180
        computer software 179
        varimax 110, 178, 180
fair treatment 28
faking *see* cheating or faking
financial considerations *see* costs
fixing the system *see* cheating or faking
focus groups 14, 102–105
follow-up 74, 77–78
forced choices, responses 120–123
frequency 157
    counts *see* tallies
    cumulative 160–161
    distribution 158–159, 167
funding *see* costs

generalisability 195
graphic scale 122
graphical representation of data 169,
    186–188
graphology 142–143, 194–195

halo effect 144–145
handouts 189
health, psychological variables 3–4

health professions, attitudes to surveys viii–x
histogram 159
human dignity 28
hypotheses
    complex 23
    deriving and formulating 18–26, 148
    not proved or disproved 25
    null 25–26
    revision 19–20
    testing 19, 57

in-depth pilot interview 100–102
incentives 74, 76
independent variables 173
indirect interviews 83
inducement *see* incentives
inexperienced researcher xi, 172
information *see* data
instant access chart xii–xiv
internet
    data entry 132
    research 57, 60–61
interruptions 101
interval scale 155, 166
interview
    costs 89
    direct and indirect 83
    length 112
    and questionnaire 87
    structured and non-structured 81, 82
    use in surveys 9, 79–82, 83–86
interviewers
    bias 90
    training and supervising 87–88
interviewing, principles 85–86
items
    analysis in opinion-based surveys 139–140
    discriminability 140
    facility 139–140
    formulation 124–125
    realistic 125
    relatedness 175

jargon 12, 100, 116, 185
justice 28

knowledge, and research 55–56

lay perceptions of health and illness (report) 235–259
    critique 259–260
letter, initial, in postal surveys 73, 75–76, 77
library research 19, 33, 56–59
line graphs 188
linear regression 173, 174
literacy, respondents 89, 189
literature review *see* library research
logical explanation 19
longitudinal designs 68–69
lying *see* cheating or faking

mail questionnaires *see* postal surveys
management
    decisions 3
    information 3, 4
    presenting information to 14, 186
Mann–Whitney U test 156, 172
mean 124, 157, 161, 162
measurement *see* scale
median 157, 161, 162–163
memory deficits 146
meta-analysis 59–60
MINITAB 180
mistakes xi, 11
mode 157, 161, 163
morale and motivation of respondents 5
multimedia techniques 189
multiple regression 173–175
multivariate statistical methods 9–10, 14

needs
    of client 13
    of respondents 6
negative correlations 169–171
negative reactions, fear of 145–146
neurological conditions, quality of life measurements 40–41
noisy surrounding 101
nominal scale 120–121, 154, 166
non-experimental descriptive design 65, 66–69
non-probability sampling 94–95
non-structured interview 80, 81, 82

Index

normal distribution 160
normative designs 66
norms 66, 68–69
null hypotheses 25–26

obesity (report) 198–234
   critique 234–235
objective criteria 5
objective evaluations 3
objective information 33
objective questions 112
objectives
   checklist 22
   clear and explicit 8, 12, 57
   client's 20–22
   determining 18–26
   and hypotheses 22–26
   inappropriate or unethical 29
observations, in survey creation 99
open questions 111, 113, 115–116
opinion-based surveys, item analysis 139–140
opportunistic sampling 94
oral presentation of report 188–190
order of questions 112–114
ordinal scale *see* rank scale
ordinary people 103
organizations
   change 7
   culture 6–7
   evaluation 5
   political dimension 49–50

p-value 181
panel designs 69
patients
   backgrounds, assessment 7
   care and treatment, evaluation 3
   discontent 14–15
Pearson product-moment correlation 156, 166, 171
percentages 157, 172
perceptions, and objective criteria 5
personal information 113–114, 117
pictures, in final report 188
pie diagrams 187
pilot study 9, 13–14, 109
   interviewing subject experts 100–102

number of respondents 138
   qualitative 137–138, 149–150
   quantitative 138–150
placebo group 70
planning 153
political dimension of surveys 49–50
population, definition 92
positive correlation 169–171
postal surveys 9, 73–79, 90
prediction 143–144, 148, 173, 174
presentation software 189
presentation of survey results 82, 185–190
privacy 28, 74
projection 146
psychological variables, in health 3–4
psychological/psychiatric morbidity, quality of life questionnaires 36–37
purposive sampling 95

qualitative approach, pilot study 137–138, 149–150
quality audits 6–7
quality of life questionnaires 34–43
quantifiable information 4
quantitative approach, pilot project 138–150
quasi-experimental design 65–66, 69–71
questionnaire
   culture-specific 68
   format 76–77
   and interview 87
   items *see* items
   language 54
   length 112, 113
   number of questions 12–13
   structuring contents 105–109
   user-friendliness 9, 12, 74
questionnaire, *see also* survey
questions
   branching 115
   closed 116–20
   logical sequence 112
   open-ended 115–116
   order 112–114

random dialling 84

randomisation 112–113
range 157, 164
rank scale 122–123, 154–155, 166, 171–172
rating errors 144–146
rating scale 121
ratio scale 155, 166
reading ability *see* literacy
recording 101, 102
recruitment and selection, assessing 6
regression 173–175
relationships or associations 156
relevance 116
reliability 140–141, 149
reminders 74
repetition, avoiding 112
report
   contents 185–186
   critiques 234–235, 259–260, 274–275
   evaluating 191–197
   examples 198–275
   focus group 103
   oral presentation 188–190
   quality 192–193
   scientific or non-scientific 193–194
   structure 191–192
   suitability for intended readership 185
representative sample, definition 92
research
   and knowledge 55–56
   need for 52–55
   theoretical rationale 57
researcher
   definition xii
   developing knowledge 55–56
   inexperienced xi, 172
   internal or external 15–17
   qualifications 15
   responsibility 132
   self-development 55
   written contract 8, 45–48
respiratory conditions, quality of life measurements 39
respondents
   acceptability of items and format 100, 116–117
   anonymity 15, 74, 78, 90, 113–114
   confidentiality 15, 48, 74, 78

   consent 28, 30
   costs 77
   definition xii
   embarrassment 125
   incentives 74, 76
   literacy 89, 189
   morale and motivation 5
   needs 6
   rights 27, 28
   vulnerable 29
response
   combining 124
   to forced choices 120–123
   numerical value 124
   rate 74–79, 90
results, presentation 9–10, *see also* report
reverse-scoring 132
rheumatological conditions, quality of life measurements 41
role functioning, psychological/psychiatric morbidity 37
rotation *see* factor rotation; varimax rotation

sample
   definition 92
   finding 95
   size 78–79, 80, 92–95, 156
sampling
   credibility 79, 93
   efficiency 84
   equal probability 93–94
   error 92
   method 9
   non-probability 94–95
   sample size and type 92–95
scale
   additive 123–124
   mid-point 123
   types 154–155
   validity 141–149
scanning, hardware and software 132
scatter-plot 167, 168, 169, 170, 171
scientific method 18–20
scores, mean 124
scree slope method 110, 179
secrecy 15, *see also* anonymity; confidentiality

Index

self-determination 28
simple random sampling 93–94
simulation studies 71
slides 189
small-group discussion, in pilot project 138
software *see* computer methods
Spearman rank-order correlation 156, 166, 171–172
speed of survey 44–45, 84, 90
sponsorship 74–76
spreadsheets 131, 180–181
SPSS 180
staff
    dissatisfaction 5, 14
    evaluation 5, 7, 30
standard deviation 157, 164–166
standard English 116, 124–125
standard error, definition 92
statistical analysis, computer methods 9, 91, 153, 154, 172, 180–181
statistical significance 181
stepwise multiple regression 174–175
stratified random sampling 94
structured interview 79, 81, 82
subgroups, differentiating 94
subject experts 100–102, 105, *see also* expert group
subjective evaluations 3
subjective questions 112
summary *see* abstract
survey
    administration methods 9, 89–91
    computer methods 82–83, 90–91
    contradictory answers 117–118
    costs 3, 14, 44, 49
    cross-sectional 156
    data analysis 153–181
    design xi, 8–9
    desirable characteristics 11–13
    drafting 107
    ethical considerations 29–31
    evaluation 140–149
    format and design 114–115
    in the health professions viii–x
    interview 79–82, 83–86
    items *see* items
    length 77, 111–122
    longitudinal 156
    multidimensional 14
    need for 31–33
    objectives *see* objectives
    off-the-shelf 8, 33–44
    order of questions 112–114
    overview of process 8–10
    piloting 9, 13–14, 109, 137–150
    political dimension 49–50
    postal administration 9, 73–79, 90
    reasons for 3–8
    reliability 140–141, 142, 189
    report *see* report
    results
        acting on 5, 10, 15, 29–30
        presentation 185–190
    speed and time considerations 44–45, 84, 90
    telephone 84–85, 89, 112
    types 112, 154–155
    validity 13, 189
    writing 111–133
survey, *see also* questionnaire
symptom scales, psychological/psychiatric morbidity 37
systematic sampling 95

t-test 156, 172, 174
    dependent 156
    paired 173
tables and graphs, use in report 186–187
tallies 156, 157–161
telephone surveys 84–85, 89, 112
terms, definition xi–xii, 92
terms and conditions *see* written contract
theory, development 100
think-tank 102
thinking aloud 137–138
time considerations 8, 44–45, 84, 90, 112
transparencies 189
trend designs 68–69
trends, measuring 173
trial run *see* pilot study
two-way frequency distribution 167

unbiased information 4–5, 84
user-friendliness 9, 12, 74

vague wording, avoiding 21
validity 141–149
variables
   dependent and independent 173
   measuring 57
variance 164–166
   analysis *see* ANOVA
variation, measures 156, 157, 163–166
varimax rotation 110, 178, 180

wording
   clarity 21
   using standard English 116, 124–125
work experience, measurements 44
working day 101
written contract, researcher 8, 45–48

yes/no responses 120